Nursing Research
An Ethical and Legal Appraisal

Edited by

Louise de Raeve

Centre for Philosophy and Health Care
University of Wales, Swansea
Singleton Park
Swansea, UK

Baillière Tindall
London Philadelphia Toronto Sydney Tokyo

Baillière Tindall   24–28 Oval Road
London NW1 7DX

The Curtis Center
Independence Square West
Philadelphia, PA 19106–3399, USA

Harcourt Brace & Company
55 Horner Avenue
Toronto, Ontario M8Z 4X6, Canada

Harcourt Brace & Company, Australia
30–52 Smidmore Street
Marrickville
NSW 2204, Australia

Harcourt Brace & Company, Japan
Ichibancho Central Building
22-1 Ichibancho
Chiyoda-ku, Tokyo 102, Japan

This book is printed on acid-free paper

A catalogue record for this book is available from the British Library

ISBN 0-7020-1888-0

Typeset by WestKey Ltd, Falmouth, Cornwall
Printed and bound in Great Britain by WBC Book Manufacturers Ltd,
Bridgend, Mid Glamorgan.

Contents

III. Broader Issues

Appendix

Contributors

Sylvia Buckingham R.S.C.N.; B.Ed (Hons); Dip. N.(London); R.N.T.: trained at Birmingham Children's Hospital and afterwards moved to Oxford where she was a staff nurse on various children's wards. In 1988 she became a nurse tutor at the John Radcliffe Hospital and in 1991 a Lecturer Practitioner, moving to Kings College Hospital in 1993 as Head of Nursing for Child Health. She has recently taken up an appointment as Lecturer in Child Health at the Nightingale Institute, Kings College London. She is currently studying for a Masters in Nursing at Kings College. Special interests include pain management and skills development in qualified nurses. **Address:** Lecturer in Social Science and Child Health, Nightingale Institute, Shepherd's House, Guy's Hospital, St Thomas' Street, London SE1 9RT.

Louise de Raeve B.A. (Hons); R.G.N.; Diploma in the Ethics of Health Care: after completing a first degree in philosophy, trained as a general nurse in the early '70's. She has since worked in a variety of settings including a therapeutic community and the voluntary sector. She moved into teaching nurses in 1989 and in her current post is the Macmillan Lecturer in Nursing Ethics at the Centre for Philosophy and Health Care, University of Wales, Swansea. **Address:** Macmillan Lecturer in Nursing Ethics, Centre for Philosophy and Health Care, University of Wales, Swansea, Singleton Park, Swansea SA2 8PP.

Bridgit Dimond M.A.; L.L.B.; D.S.A.; A.H.S.M.; Barrister-at-Law: is a former health service manager, lecturer and Assistant Director of the University of Glamorgan. She is currently Chairman of the Mid Glamorgan Family Health Services Authority and was a member of the Mental Health Act Commission. Bridgit Dimond is author of "Legal Aspects of Nursing" (Prentice Hall 2nd edition 1995) and "Legal Aspects of Midwifery" (Books for Midwives Press 1994) and numerous articles on health service law. She is currently Emeritus Professor of the University of Glamorgan. **Address:** Emeritus Professor, University of Glamorgan, Pontypridd, Mid Glamorgan CF37 1DL.

Steven Ersser R.G.N.; B.Sc. (Hons): has been involved in a variety of clinical roles including those which combine practice development and research. Until recently he was a Fellow of the National Institute for Nursing, Radcliffe Infirmary N.H.S. Trust, Oxford. He is now Senior Lecturer and Research Associate in the School of Health Care Studies, Oxford Brookes University, with a specific responsibility for research and post-graduate courses in advanced health care practice. **Address:** Senior Lecturer/Research Associate, School of Health Care Studies, Oxford Brookes University, Academic Centre, John Radcliffe Hospital, Headington, Oxford OX3 9DU.

Barbara Johnson S.R.N.; Dip. in Community Nursing; H.V. Cert.; Q.N.; Teaching Cert.; Ph.D.: spent several years in health and cancer education before moving into social research. She has worked on a number of projects concerned mainly with the psychosocial implications of cancer prevention and cancer management. This has involved accessing and in-depth interviewing of both health professionals and the lay public. Barbara Johnson is currently a lecturer in the Department of Nursing Studies at King's College London. **Address:** Department of Nursing Studies, King's College London, Waterloo Road, London.

Judith Lathlean B.Sc. (Econ); M.A.; D.Phil.: is a social scientist by background and has considerable experience of undertaking and managing nursing, health care and education research. Until recently, she was the Director of the G.N.C. Trust Nurse Education Research Unit at the University of Surrey. She is now an independent research consultant, educator and writer and is also visiting Professor at the University of Surrey and at the University of Reading. **Address:** Judith Lathlean, Research Associates Cedar Cottage, North Side, Steeple Aston, Bicester, Oxfordshire OX6 3SE.

Kim Lützén R.N.; PhD: has been a psychiatric nurse for many years and is currently Senior Lecturer and Chair of the Department of Nursing, Stockholm University College and a researcher at the Ersta Institute of Health Care Ethics, Stockholm. Her current interest is researching into ethical problems and moral reasoning using qualitative methodology. **Address:** RN Associate Professor, Health Care Ethics, Ersta University College, Institute of Health Care Ethics, Box 4619, S11691, Stockholm, Sweden.

Donna Mead R.G.N.; M.Sc.; Ph.D.; R.N.T.: is Head of Research and Development and Graduate Studies in a large Department of Nursing, Midwifery and Health Care. She oversees the research component of all courses and co-ordinates the Research Degree programme. In 1991, out of ethical concern she called for a moratorium on all nursing research below Masters level. **Address:** Assistant Director, Department of Nursing, Midwifery and Health

Care, University of Wales, Swansea, Singleton Park, Swansea SA2 8PP.

Neil Pickering B.A.; M.A.; M.Phil.: worked as a Research Assistant on the Centre for Philosophy and Health Care (CPHC) reports to the Department of Health entitled 'The Conduct of Ethical Review of Multi-Location Research' and 'The Training Needs of Members of Local Research Ethics Committees'. He is on the current teaching faculty for AICRC/CPHC Training Conference for members of Research Ethics Committees and is a University College Fellow in the CPHC, University of Wales, Swansea. **Address:** Centre for Philosophy and Health Care, University of Wales, Swansea, Singleton Park, Swansea SA2 8PP.

Hilary Plant R.G.N.; B.A.: trained and worked as a cancer nurse before reading history at the London School of Economics. She is currently completing her Ph.D. at King's College London and is a part-time lecturer at the Centre for Cancer and Palliative Care Studies at the Royal Marsden Hospital and Institute of Cancer Research. Her interests include the impact of cancer on the family and qualitative research methods. **Address:** Lecturer in Cancer Nursing, Academic Nursing Unit, Royal Marsden Hospital, Fulham Road, London SW3.

Jill Rogers B.A.; M.Phil.: has considerable experience in research in continuing professional education having managed projects for the Department of Health and the English National Board. She is Director of Jill Rogers Associates, a consultancy committed to providing quality project management in health care and related professions. **Address:** Jill Rogers Associates, 2 Flint Bridge Business Centre, Ely Road, White Beach, Cambridgeshire, CB5 9PG.

Roger Watson B.Sc.; Ph.D.; R.G.N.; C.Biol.; M.I. Biol.: originally studied and researched in biochemistry at the Universities of Edinburgh and Sheffield. He moved into nursing and worked in Care of the Elderly as a Staff Nurse and as a Charge Nurse. He currently lectures at the University of Edinburgh. **Address:** Senior Lecturer, Department of Nursing Studies, The University of Edinburgh, Edinburgh, EH8 9LL.

Introduction

In 1991, I had reason to investigate the literature on the ethics of nursing research and I was surprised to find there was relatively little written on the subject. The only comprehensive book that I could find was one edited by Anne Davis and Janette Krueger (1980) which was out of print. Noting what seemed to me to be a need and a lack of material to meet it, I decided to contact some possible contributors and present a proposal.

In the course of this enterprise, it was immensely encouraging to find that not only were some nurse–researchers willing to write a chapter, they were positively eager to do so. They felt that the dilemmas they had struggled with in relative isolation needed sharing so that mistakes might not be repeated by the unwary and so that inevitable and sometimes insoluble moral difficulties could at least be anticipated and planned for.

Ethics cannot be seen simply as an analysis of when one gets it right and when one makes mistakes for this would presuppose shared agreement about what is 'right' and what is 'wrong'. We all understand the concepts but may disagree about their use in particular instances since different people often evaluate the same event differently. Fundamentalist religious traditions, for example, would assert that there is an independent source for establishing moral answers but in cultures of moral pluralism, it seems a widely held view that there is no such ultimate 'court of appeal'. Therefore, whilst it is of the utmost importance to argue and seek to persuade others and one may be successful, there always remains the possibility that some moral disagreements will prove to be insoluble. Some see this as a cause for celebration rather than dismay and this would be a liberal, democratic view.

A personal moral dilemma occurs when moral tension is found within one individual rather than between two people. In such a predicament one feels deeply torn, knowing that whatever one chooses to do there are compelling arguments for deciding differently. Inevitably, one feels less than virtuous in such circumstances, although one may accept that one made the best decision one could.

Many of the first seven chapters in this book record instances of this type where the pull to be a good nurse is in very painful tension with the pull to be a good researcher. To proceed with both aims inevitably results in compromises about which people feel less than happy. It is to be hoped that readers will respect the fact that many authors in this book have written with courage, taking the risk to describe events and behaviour that they themselves feel troubled about.

I make no claim that these ethical difficulties could ever be resolved. However, it does seem imperative that as a profession we discuss these issues together, to enable us to come to some professional agreement about what degree of tension should be tolerated and at what point the researcher role should be relinquished in favour of care and vice-versa. This debate clearly needs to take place within nursing but also I think it needs to take place with patients. There are of course immense difficulties in trying to find truly representative and cohesive groups of patients or ex-patients who could be approached in this way. Nevertheless, it seems important to try since these are the people who, if anyone does, have a stake in both receiving good nursing care and an interest in promoting research which will improve it. What kind of research do patients want us to conduct and what can they tolerate? In the highly politicised world of AIDS and HIV research these questions had to be asked and answered since more conventional approaches had foundered: the subversive (from the research perspective) activities of patients desperate to receive medication were invalidating the data (Nairne, 1992).

It is hoped that the sequence of contents in the book will be attractive to readers and inviting both to those who may prefer the story of experiences from which they can draw their own conclusions and to those who wish to combine this with a more analytic approach. **Section I** consists of seven chapters written for the most part by nurse–researchers. These describe the ethical issues which the researcher faced while doing a particular piece of research. Two chapters in this section have been written by non-nurses who have made a career in research and specialised in using the methods they describe. Both have spent a considerable period of their research life researching into nurses and nursing and might, therefore, qualify as honorary nurses. An attempt has been made to cover all the basic methods of research: experimental, survey, action research and the ethnographic case study approach. Inevitably not all techniques are considered, for example, the Delphi method is not examined at all.

In addition to method and technique, an attempt has been made to consider a range of research amongst different patient populations. Chapter 1 examines research in elderly care where many patients were demented and thus could not give informed consent. Chapter 5 describes research in a paediatric ward, Chapter 6 is located in a psychiatric unit and Chapter 7 focuses on research with people who have cancer. Again, it is not possible to cover everything and no particular mention is made of research with people with learning difficulties, with the criminally insane or in the field of midwifery. However, readers from these specialities should still find plenty to interest them in this book since similar issues will undoubtedly occur in their own contexts, albeit with different slants of meaning and degrees of emphasis. Indeed on reading Chapters 1–7 one cannot help being struck by the similarity of many of the concerns raised. For this reason the ethical commentary has been reserved for Chapter 8, thereby permitting comparisons and contrasts to be made by drawing upon the material of all the preceding chapters.

Four out of the first seven chapters explore research which focuses on nurses rather than patients. This is a bias in the book which has emerged rather than been deliberately sought and it must, I think, reflect a current professional preoccupation with the identity of nursing. Assuming that this bias is symptomatic of a wider tendency, the issue could again be profitably discussed within the profession. Have we got the balance right between looking at what nurses do and think, and research that is directed primarily at discovering and understanding what nursing patients need?

Section II consists of three chapters which present an overview of the subject of nursing research and to greater or lesser degrees provide commentaries on the preceding seven chapters. It may therefore be preferable if readers read this section in sequence, having first perused the earlier chapters.

Section III of the book is more free-standing than Section II and the two chapters; one on Ethical Review and the other on Teaching Nursing and Midwifery Research could be read either in sequence or alone.

It is impossible to predict how wide-ranging the readership of this book will be. Readers should therefore be aware that whilst much of the experiential and analytic content of the chapters will be relevant to any nursing culture which conducts research, the Legal Issues chapter (Chapter 9) and the Ethical Review chapter (Chapter 11) are weighted towards the situation in England.

The level of ethical analysis is aimed at the needs of the nurse-researcher rather than towards those who have studied health care ethics in some depth. For this reason, the language is deliberately ordinary and no particular references have been made to moral theories such as utilitarianism or to moral perspectives such as duties, virtues, rights and consequences. Nevertheless, features of these perspectives are implicit in much of what is said. Moral concerns about the ambiguity of the nurse–researcher role immediately raise questions of coercion in relation to informed consent, thereby introducing the possibility that patient autonomy is compromised in some way, not just by illness but by who the nurse–researcher is perceived to be. This could be formulated as a concern about both the proper obligations of the nurse–researcher and a concern about protecting patient rights. Similarly, the exploration of means and ends in relation to research can be framed in terms of a tension between a Kantian view of the proper way of treating people (never *merely* as a means) and a utilitarian view that the size of the benefit to be gained wins the argument, regardless of the means to be used (the greatest happiness of the greatest number). These issues can, however, all be discussed without having to give them a particular historical or philosophical context and this is the preferred approach for this book. Moral analysis at a normative level is not the prerogative of the moral philosopher, it is an ordinary feature of everyday life.

Similarly, those readers who are familiar with 'ethical frameworks' may be puzzled not to find mention of them in this book. Their omission reflects a position on the matter which needs some explanation. The "principles" approach of, for example, Beauchamp and Childress (1994) is clearly a popular and for many, a helpful way of thinking about moral problems. However, in so far as all frameworks structure thought, they may both limit and facilitate it. My own preference is to avoid explicit reference to theoretical structures but inevitably this leaves me open to the objection that I have rejected a well established method of analysis. Ultimately, the wisdom of doing so is a matter of opinion about which there is no general agreement in the field of health care ethics.

Lastly, it is hoped that this book will be not only informative and thought provoking but also enjoyable to read. Perhaps due to the nature of the subject there has been considerable consultation with chapter writers in order to facilitate the integration of material. Having said this, however, it needs to be noted that Chapters 8, 9 and 10 express the views of their writers only and are not to be considered as a collective voice of other contributors to the book.

It remains for me to thank Cancer Relief Macmillan Fund who fund my post, all the contributors to the book and my colleagues in the Centre for Philosophy & Health Care (University of Wales, Swansea), most notably Neil Pickering and Martyn Evans who provided helpful criticism. Acknowledgement is also due to The World Medical Association for their permission as authors to reproduce The Helsinki Declaration as an appendix.

References

Beauchamp, T.L. and Childress, J.F. (1994) *Principles of Biomedical Ethics*, 4th edition. New York: Oxford University Press.

Davis, A.J. and Krueger, J.C. eds. (1980) *Patients, Nurses, Ethics*. New York: American Journal of Nursing Co.

Nairne, P. The Right Hon. Chairman of I.M.E. Working Party on the ethical implications of AIDS. (1992) AIDS, ethics, and clinical trials. *British Medical Journal* **305**, 19th September pp. 699–701.

I

Research Experiences

1

Product Testing on Trial

Roger Watson

Introduction

Product testing is something in which nurses are always involved. In whatever speciality they work, technology is continually improving the equipment which is used for patient care, and nurses are expected to implement this equipment in practice. Sometimes they are asked their opinion about the equipment but, often, they are not.

The pressure to integrate new equipment into patient care is high. New staff arrive from other areas and newly trained staff arrive from the colleges of nursing. In both areas these staff will have been exposed to different types of equipment and may have better ideas about what can be used. Sales representatives constantly vie for contracts with local budget holders. In many cases, senior nurses are approached and may be impressed by something which is not currently in use in their areas of clinical responsibility. Another pressure, not necessarily based on any notions of improvement, may be purely financial (Farmer and Watson, 1989). Again, such pressure may come from budget holders and the pressure in this case may be to try something new because it is cheaper. It is not necessarily appropriate to expound in this chapter the reasons why a piece of equipment may be cheaper. This may result purely from a "sales pitch" to gain access to a health authority or clinical directorate; the equipment may, indeed, be cheaper – it may be better. However, it will often be the case that, based on what is presented by sales representatives or by local budget holders, the nurse working in the clinical area – the ward manager (sister or charge nurse) will have very little information on which to base a decision and, possibly, very little influence over the final choice of equipment (Watson, 1989a).

Equipment

The term "equipment" covers a multitude of items and aids used in nursing. In the present chapter it is meant to represent appliances over which nurses have the major say regarding implementation with individual patients. Such devices include absorbent pads and a variety of external drainage devices. It is such equipment, for the management of urinary incontinence, which forms the basis of the work described in this chapter.

Urinary Incontinence

Urinary incontinence, while its prevalence definitely increases with age, is not an inevitable part of the ageing process. Nevertheless, the prevalence of urinary incontinence in both sexes increases with age (Thomas *et al.*, 1986) and is associated with the kind of frailty and impairment which causes admission to many continuing care of the elderly settings. Indeed, urinary incontinence is often sufficient reason for admittance of a frail elderly person to a continuing care setting (Palmer, 1988).

Nurses have a major responsibility, especially in institutional settings, for the management of urinary incontinence (Hall *et al.*, 1993). It is not surprising, therefore, that a major part of the nursing workload and effort in planning the delivery of care in such settings is concerned with the alleviation and, where possible, the prevention of urinary incontinence. The problems of urinary incontinence for individual patients are manifold and include discomfort, odour, skin excoriation (Watson, 1993), psychological withdrawal and social isolation (Grimby *et al.*, 1993) and damage to clothing. Where the urinary incontinence cannot be prevented, and this chapter is not the place to debate the issue of prevention versus alleviation, it is necessary to minimise the problems associated with incontinence for individual patients. The use of equipment is always controversial but, where it is to be used, it can be done with success if individual patients are carefully selected for use with specific pieces of equipment (Norton, 1987). The choice of equipment should be based, wherever possible, on research data and, where this is not available, the possibility of testing equipment arises. It is the testing of such equipment in a continuing care of the elderly setting, where the majority of patients were suffering from dementia, that will be described below.

Background to the Studies

The work described here was carried out at Kirklandside Hospital in Kilmarnock between 1987 and 1989. This was one of the many periods of great upheaval in the Health Service and the particular upheaval which was taking place at that time was the introduction of devolved budgeting. I would not like to suggest that nurses working in this, or any other area of the Health Service were unconcerned about the products which they were using with their patients before this time. However, the concept of devolved budgeting pushed accountability for spending closer to the points at which care was being delivered and, therefore, the point at which equipment was being used. This could be viewed as a positive development (Watson, 1992). This provided a stimulus and the opportunity to many, including clinical nurse managers and charge nurses, to look closely at the equipment they were using and decide if it could be used more cost-effectively or if alternative equipment could be used.

The concept of cost-effectiveness

Cost-effectiveness is one of the most elusive concepts in any area and especially in health care (Watson, 1990). It is frequently the case that those who consider the concept have conflicting aims and objectives, albeit not expressed, and therefore have different ideas of what cost-effectiveness means. Taking the example of the equipment used in the management of urinary incontinence, the person who is actually accountable for the budget at unit level may be presented with the possibility of purchasing two alternatives. One alternative may be cheaper per unit cost (i.e. cost per item) than the other. In other words, supplying a ward with the normal quota of equipment for the management of urinary incontinence may be much cheaper if, say, one type of absorbent pad or one type of urinary sheath is bought rather than another. On the other hand, at the ward level the least expensive alternative may not be as easy to use and may require more to be used per patient. It can be difficult, even if large amounts of equipment requiring large amounts of money are being used at ward level, to effect a change in purchasing policy. To the person with ultimate control over the budget, it probably appears logical to spend the budget on that which appears to be cheaper.

Product testing

At Kirklandside Hospital the clinical nurse manager* was particularly keen to achieve cost-effectiveness – in the correct sense of the term, i.e. to spend money wisely and also to achieve a high standard of patient care. In order to achieve this the charge nurses were made aware of their individual ward budgets and encouraged to look at patient care. One particular area of high spending, in this continuing care setting, was on equipment for the manage-

* Dr Elizabeth Farmer, currently Reader at Highland College of Nursing and Midwifery, Inverness.

ment of urinary incontinence. This was particularly the case on the male ward where urinary sheaths were commonly used; these have a high unit cost relative to other items such as absorbent pads and questions were therefore raised about spending on those particular items. Simultaneously, representatives from commercial companies who manufactured both urinary sheaths and absorbent pads were inviting the unit to test their products. Several commercial companies were involved in the product testing. Each company was made aware of the testing and of which rival products were being tested and was assured that it would be given the results at the earliest opportunity. The companies offered help in a number of ways by either providing free equipment for the trials or equipment at a reduced cost.

The staff at Kirklandside Hospital took up this challenge and decided to carry out systematic tests (termed "nursing trials" in order to make the comparison but also the distinction from the better known "clinical trial") of the existing products against some of the alternative products. Obviously, the trials were designed to subject all of the products to equal testing, as far as it was possible to design for this and to allow for this in the local budget. For instance, it was necessary for the ward to pay for part of some products in order to test them against products which were being provided free of charge.

Obviously, all of the companies involved expressed total confidence in their products and believed that they would have nothing to lose and everything to gain by cooperating in the trials. Our response was to ensure that they all understood that we were intending to publish the outcome of the trials and that the research was being conducted primarily for the benefit of patients and to increase nursing knowledge. In fact, we decided that we were going to proceed with the trials whether the commercial companies helped us by providing equipment or not. We had already decided which of a range of products we wished to test and felt morally obliged to proceed and to find the money from the local budget. We were, nevertheless, grateful for the involvement of the companies and never felt under any pressure to conduct the trials in any way other than according to our own design.

Ethical and Methodological Considerations

The concept of a test or trial involving patients immediately raises ethical issues. There is a kind of "uncertainty principle" at work here whereby the more ethical you try to be, the less scientific you become and getting the balance right between the two was one of the main problems of the work which will be described below.

A trial in the clinical setting is designed to test at least two alternatives. The ultimate trial, familiar to those involved in testing drugs, involves the comparison of a treatment against no treatment in order to clearly demonstrate the effectiveness (or the lack of effectiveness) of the treatment under consideration. The concept of the classical clinical trial whereby a drug is tested against no drug in the form of a placebo or simply no treatment is, however, fraught with ethical problems (le Roux, 1988a). Such a trial involves a measure of deceit towards those taking part. Needless to say, such trials should not take place without the appropriate information being given to those involved, but deceit is operated nevertheless. The individual does not know whether or not they are being treated and withholding treatment from one group may, in fact, prove to be deleterious. Moreover, the treatment under consideration may be of dubious benefit or even harmful through unknown side-effects. There are many variations on the clinical trial but any effort to increase their ethical content by, for instance, switching patients to the treatment if it proves effective and withdrawing patients mid-trial when the treatment seems to be deleterious, lessens the scientific validity of the trial. The latter is an inescapable fact of clinical trials. It is, of course, possible to compare two or more treatments without withholding treatment from one group of patients. This is described as a quasi-experiment (to distinguish it from the true experiment described above) and it proceeds without a true control group (Polit and Hungler, 1987). This also lessens the scientific validity as assumptions are made that the "treatment control" is beneficial, and any apparent improvement as a result of the treatment being tested offers a real improvement to patients over no treatment.

Designs for testing products

It was clear to us at Kirklandside Hospital that the true experiment, as represented by the classical clinical trial, was not appropriate for the studies we were about to undertake. It was evident that the use of absorbent pads and urinary sheaths was beneficial for many patients as, to some extent, they offered an improvement over totally withdrawing the use of such equipment. It was not possible, therefore, to test any products against the use of no product as this was bound to lead to a deterioration in nursing care for many of our patients. In terms of lessening the wetting of clothes, reducing odour and preventing skin excoriation, any absorbent pad, however poor its properties, or any urinary sheath, despite its tendency to become detached sooner or later, was bound to be better than leaving patients with no protection. We were not, therefore, embarking on this research in order to provide new knowledge about the management of urinary incontinence *per se*; rather, the aim was to compare products which we already knew offered some advantage to patients. We could, however, provide new knowledge about the relative effectiveness of different products.

We were aware, nevertheless, that some products offered next to no advantage to certain individual patients. For example, in some men urinary sheaths become detached very quickly for anatomical reasons or, due to confusion, they remove them. This has provided urinary sheaths, generally, with a very "bad press" (Gonsalkovale and Lawless, 1987). The same applies to the use of absorbent pads in both males and females.

It is true to say that the misuse of equipment for the management of urinary incontinence is often worse than using nothing. While such misuse of equipment may provide nurses with a false sense of security – through satisfying the natural nursing urge to "do something" – they may make the situation worse due to the fact that the equipment fails to serve its purpose. Ultimately, it allows urine to come in contact with the skin, while the patients remain unattended and at very high risk of excoriation of skin and damage to clothing by incontinent urine. We decided, therefore, to monitor the individual patients who were involved in the trials very closely in order to see which of these were most suitable for the use of urinary sheaths. Basically, those who keep the sheath *in situ* for longest, without any dermatological problems, are the ones who are most suitable. We hoped, by this means to develop an individual assessment procedure for other patients, and the outcome of this is described below.

Literature review

It could be considered unethical to proceed with any kind of research involving patients, if the researcher is not absolutely certain why the research is being carried out. Certainly, the individual researcher, or group of researchers in the clinical area may not know what the answer is to their particular problems or how to satisfy legitimate curiosity about aspects of the care which they deliver. Proceeding with research purely on the basis of such "hunches" and "fancies", however, is not justified unless the researcher, at the very least, can satisfy others that the research is worth doing and that the information which is being sought is not available elsewhere. For these reasons, a search of the available literature in the proposed field of study is mandatory, as it is only against the background of previous research and published knowledge that a research project can be proposed and implemented. With the availability of computerised databases and helpful, knowledgeable librarians in most medical and nursing libraries, there is really no excuse for not carrying out this exercise thoroughly and effectively.

In the specific case of research into equipment for the management of urinary incontinence, there was a genuine paucity of research-based publications on its use and very little evidence of systematic testing which could really guide practice or provide new knowledge. There were quite a number of publications expressing opinions about the use of equipment for the management of urinary incontinence generally but these opinions were usually only supported by anecdote. The few trials which had been published were of a very poor standard regarding control over extraneous variables or methods which accounted for these variables and which enabled sound data analysis and statistically significant conclusions to be drawn.

Justification for Research Design

The trials reported here were designed to test the relative effectiveness of a number of urinary sheaths, urine collecting bags and absorbent disposable pads for the management of irreversible urinary incontinence. A general discussion of some of the principles involved in the design of product testing trials has been given above and it is the purpose of this section to specifically describe and justify the design used in the trials reported here.

Quasi-experimental crossover trials

The design used was quasi-experimental in that control groups of subjects were not used (Polit and Hungler, 1987). As previously described, this would not have been feasible for the testing of products, examples of which were already in use at the time of the trials. A crossover design was used whereby all of the participants in the trial used all of the products tested at some point in the trial. For the purpose of data analysis, the data for all of the products as used by all individuals are "pooled" and form the basis of the statistical testing to ascertain effectiveness.

The crossover design has many features, most of which are positive, which militated in favour of its use in the present trials. The classical clinical trial design divides subjects into two groups and, as described above, one group is treated and the other is not (or an existing treatment is applied). Notwithstanding the procedures for the selection of subjects such as random selection followed by random allocation to treatment or non-treatment groups, which are designed to avoid systematic error, there are significant problems in obtaining a truly random sample. Usually, some compromise is made by the use of convenience samples or random selection within a very narrow cluster of potential subjects. The absence of true randomness in the selection of subjects limits the extent to which results can be generalised (le Roux, 1988b). The crossover design minimises the effect of differences between subjects by exposing all subjects to the alternatives of treatment or non-treatment at some point throughout the period of the trial (Beck, 1989). Another advantageous feature of the crossover design is that it reduces the number of subjects required in order to test treatments compared with group comparison, as the subjects can be used for both treatment and non-treatment testing. Nevertheless, the time of the trial may have to be extended in order to accommodate this testing of treatment and non-treatment, and this leads to the major disadvantage of the crossover design.

While individual variation at any point in time is reduced by the crossover design, the variation between individuals over time is not; individuals may deteriorate over the period of the trial and, depending upon the order in which products are tested, this can influence the results. The systematic element to such error in crossover designs can be minimised by random allocation, which is a minimum requirement in any trial of treatments. However, the most deleterious outcome of the variation-over-time factor is withdrawal from the trial through death or voluntary reasons. This immediately leads to a loss of subject data from whatever period in the trial they were involved. The classical clinical trial, using large groups, does not suffer to the same extent from this, as it is possible to take inequality between group numbers into account in the statistical analysis (Carriere, 1994).

Clinical consideration in crossover designs

The above considerations are mainly methodological. While they have both theoretical and practical significance, there is one aspect of the crossover design which is important clinically. The fact that all of the subjects are used to test all of the appliances in the process of the trial means that individual suitability to particular pieces of equipment can be gauged. Moreover, the general suitability of subjects for such equipment can also be gauged by analysing general aspects of the performance of equipment with individuals. It is possible, therefore, to investigate differences between individuals as well as differences between pieces of equipment. Thus our aim of making these investigations "nursing trials", whereby individuals would undergo assessment for equipment for the management of urinary incontinence, was achieved.

Recruitment of subjects

The recruitment of subjects into the trials which are described here raised several issues. It should be emphasised, however, that the problem was not one of locating suitable subjects – which is the main problem with many trials. Rather, it was the problem of ensuring that the subjects which we had in mind, i.e. those patients under our care, could be recruited in a way that was ethically justifiable. At the outset to this section I should make it clear that neither informed consent from patients nor informed consent by proxy was sought, and it is my intention to make it clear why we felt it was justified to proceed under such circumstances.

All of the subjects recruited into the trials described here were patients at Kirklandside Hospital. At any particular time, only a small number of patients were involved in a trial. For instance, the urinary sheath trials were conducted using only six subjects. However, these subjects had repeated fittings of the urinary sheaths over a three-week period, and the outcome of the trial was judged, as described below, according to the comparison of the performance of sheaths across these multiple fittings.

These patients were very "available" and we had to assure ourselves that it was not simply their availability which was driving us to conduct the trials. The majority of patients in this hospital suffered from some degree of cognitive impairment and many had the diagnosis of dementia. A high proportion were in the advanced stages of different types of dementia, including Alzheimer's disease and multi-infarct dementia. There was a range, therefore, of cognitive abilities and, concomitantly, a range of ability to understand what recruitment into the trials meant.

The normal procedure in any trial is to seek the informed consent of the individual who is being recruited into the trial, and this means that they are informed about the nature of the trial, including any potential risks to which they may be exposed. Their consent to involvement is then sought – with the provision that they may withdraw at any point – either in writing, by means of a signature, or merely verbally, in which case the researcher is satisfied that the person understands the nature of the research and is willing to participate (Royal College of Physicians, 1990).

In cases where it is impossible to obtain informed consent, where the person is either too young or mentally incapacitated to understand the nature of the research, it is standard practice to obtain informed consent by proxy (Royal College of Physicians, 1990). This means that some person who is thought to be able to represent the incapable person is informed about the research and their consent to involvement of the person is sought either verbally or in writing.

Problems with informed consent by proxy

Many problems are raised, however, by informed consent by proxy and, in the context of the trials described here, there are additional problems. These will be considered in turn.

Informed consent by proxy, despite its common application in research involving human subjects, does not really eradicate ethical problems. Rather, it serves mainly to conform to standard practice and, possibly, to ease the conscience of the researcher. These are strong words indeed, but they are borne out in the literature (Melnick *et al.*, 1984). Except in the case of children, where most traditions and legal systems accept that parents are truly able to represent the best interests of the child, it is not possible (and not logical) that anyone can really take a decision on behalf of another.

It can never really be ascertained, in the case of a mentally incompetent adult, what their wishes would really be under a given set of circumstances (Watson, 1994). It is beyond the scope of this chapter, but worth mentioning in passing, that this severely limits the kind of research in which adults who are mentally incapable can be involved. Essentially, the only kind of research in which they can be involved is the evaluation of treatments aimed at alleviating the problems from which they suffer (McCall Smith, 1992). In short, it is not ethically possible, despite informed consent by proxy, for instance, to involve elderly people with dementia in clinical trials of drugs which are not being tested for their ability to treat dementia.

The possibility of advanced consent to involvement in research has been raised with the additional possibility of indicating in advance which types of research an individual would or would not wish to be involved in (Melnick *et al.*, 1984). However, there are recorded cases of individuals with dementia being recruited, by means of informed consent by proxy, into research which it was known they would not have wished to be involved in (Warren *et al.*, 1986). The above is meant to illustrate, therefore, that there are real ethical problems with informed consent by proxy in the recruitment of elderly people with dementia into research and that researchers in this area should not hide behind this alone as an ethical justification for the involvement of such subjects.

Specific to the present work, which involved elderly patients with dementia, was that the trials included existing products, for which the use with individual patients had never been consented to. The use of such products and, indeed, most aspects of nursing and many aspects of medical care, simply proceeded on the principle of best interests and the assumption that, if the individual was able to give consent, they would wish the treatment to be applied (Watson, 1992). This is the normal state of affairs in the care of elderly people with dementia. As an example, it would be unreasonable to expect to seek consent for the alleviation of pain by pharmacological means where this increased the comfort of the patient, any more than it would be necessary to seek specific consent for regular hygiene measures despite the fact that individuals may not understand any of these aspects of care and may, in fact, offer some resistance to their implementation.

The nub of the ethical problem in the trials reported here was that products which had never been tested before were being introduced and that they were, in every sense of the word, being tested. Nevertheless, the principle of using such equipment was not being tested. Therefore, as it would be difficult to contest the continued use of existing products with these patients, it could also be viewed as ethically justified to introduce new products, even if these were being tested. It was the experience of the nurses who conducted the trials that many new products were introduced without any consent being sought and, in fact, it was the periodic introduction of new products which stimulated these trials to be carried out. This took place as a result of changes in purchasing policies at a district level whereby the purchase of one product was stopped and an alternative – usually offering some financial gain – was introduced.

It can be seen, therefore, that seeking consent under these circumstances did not appear to be necessary to the nurses who were conducting the trials, and the local research ethics committee agreed with this and allowed the trials to proceed without specific consent. This was the case for all of the reasons outlined above. Naturally, no patients who were not currently managed for urinary incontinence by means of the equipment described here, were involved in testing.

A further support for the way in which the testing was carried out came from the United Kingdom Central Council on Nursing, Midwifery and Health Visiting (1989) document on accountability which made the suggestion that limited research which was specifically aimed at improving the care of patients who were unable to give consent could be carried out. The UKCC document pointed out that the need to gain consent of any kind with such patients could preclude conducting any kind of nursing research with such patients.

With patients who had some residual cognitive skills, and who were currently using equipment to manage urinary incontinence, we did explain that some new equipment was being tested. The days on which the trials were being conducted were designated "research days" by means of notices in the ward and at the beds of those patients involved in the trials. Thus the relatives who visited were aware of the trials and any questions which they had were answered by nursing staff. We did consider asking consent from the individuals who could understand and from relatives of those who could not understand but who visited regularly. This, however, would not have solved the problem of those who could not understand and who did not have regular, if any, visitors. We felt that to use selective consent in this way would be to discriminate in favour of those patients who were fortunate enough to have residual cognitive skills and privileged enough to have regular visitors.

Conducting the Trials

Three nursing trials were conducted at Kirklandside between 1988 and 1989 in which products used for the management of urinary incontinence were tested. These trials will be outlined below and the results will be presented briefly. All of the work has been published and the relevant publications are referred to.

Urinary sheaths

Two trials were conducted on the male ward at Kirklandside and both of these were designed to test urinary sheath systems. The first trial (Watson, 1989b) was designed to test three competing systems, two of which were used as they were supplied by the manufacturing companies, i.e. with the sheath and the drainage bag both made by the same manufacturer, and the third system was a hybrid where it was necessary to incorporate a type of drainage bag for which no specific sheath was supplied. The second trial (Watson and Kuhn, 1990) was designed to test the performance of different components of the urinary sheath systems. As indicated above, each trial only used six subjects from the ward and these subjects were randomly selected from the available subjects who were using urinary sheaths at the time of the trial. A random selection of subjects was made for each trial, therefore the actual group of patients involved in each of the trials was not the same. The units of data used for statistical analysis were the lengths of time for which the urinary sheaths remained *in situ*. Throughout the trials the penile skin condition of the subjects was rigorously monitored on a daily basis with the provision being made that the subjects would be withdrawn from the trials if their skin condition deteriorated to greater than grade II in depth, according to a standard pressure sore grading system (Shea, 1975). The total number of fittings, therefore, was sufficient for statistical analysis, by analysis of variance in the first trial and *t*-test in the second. Each system was fitted 42 times to the subjects in the first trial and 30 times in the second trial, according to the crossover design outlined above.

Results of urinary sheath trials

One system was found to perform better than the other two in the first trial. The difference in performance was statistically significant and it was also considered to be clinically significant as the best system remained *in situ* for an average time which was greater than the length of time which the patients spent out of bed. This meant that, on average, the sheath would keep clothing dry, obviate patient discomfort and reduce nursing workload. Moreover, during the trial, it was not found necessary in any of the subjects (and this applied to the second trial) to withdraw them from the investigation. A very strict protocol for the fitting of sheaths and the care of skin was implemented during the trials and this was a major spin-off for clinical practice.

We had shown that it was possible, contrary to the opinion of some nurses in our area, to use urinary sheaths safely and effectively. The protocol was then adopted permanently. The possibility that components of the systems rather than the whole systems may be responsible for the performance of systems was raised after the first trial and, by using different combinations of components, this was tested in the second trial. It was, indeed, demonstrated that, while one urinary sheath was superior to another, it was also the case that one drainage bag increased the performance of both urinary sheaths. The outcome of this was that a combined system was then purchased and used.

Finally, the results from individual subjects involved in the trials were analysed after the trials and it was shown that for some individuals, urinary sheath systems did not remain *in situ* for appropriate lengths of time. It was shown that five days of fitting, taking the average length of time for which a sheath remained *in situ* were sufficient to demonstrate this in individuals. This led to a protocol being developed for the assessment of individuals for whom the management of urinary incontinence was desired. If individuals could not tolerate a urinary sheath then some alternative system, such as absorbent pads, was implemented.

In summary, therefore, we considered that we had reached several objectives in achieving our aim of carrying out the above trials. We had tested alternative systems and shown that, as they were presented by the manufacturers, it was possible to detect differences in performance; we had provided new knowledge about components of systems and their influence on overall performance; by demonstrating that urinary sheath systems could be used safely we were able to implement a protocol for their use in clinical practice and we were able to implement a protocol for assessing individuals for suitability for urinary sheath systems. Furthermore, with reference to cost-effectiveness, it was demonstrated that the system with the highest unit cost (i.e. cost per item) was the cheapest to use because, due to the length of time for which it remained *in situ*, it required the use of fewer pieces of equipment. The absorbent pad trial (Buchan and Watson, 1991) conducted on one of the female wards at Kirklandside Hospital produced a similar kind of result: the more expensive pad performed better and was thus judged to be more cost-effective.

Conclusion

The successful outcome of these trials has been described above, and those involved would certainly recommend the use of this design. There are, undoubtedly, limitations; among these are the fact that it is virtually impossible (and certainly was not attempted in the above trials) to introduce any element of "blindness" in assessing the use of equipment for the management of urinary incontinence. The results should be viewed in this light. Also, the comfort of the systems for the individuals involved and any other subjective aspects of their use cannot be gauged as, in almost all cases, the patients involved in these trials were severely cognitively impaired. Ethical questions remain, therefore, but in all of the work reported here, the trials were testing equipment which was intended for use in conditions which the patients involved actually suffered from. This is an absolute requirement in any research work involving elderly people with dementia.

References

Beck, S.L. (1989) The crossover design in clinical nursing research. *Nursing Research*, **38**, 291–293.

Buchan, R. and Watson, R. (1991) A nursing trial of absorbent disposable incontinence pads. *Care of the Elderly*, **3**(2), 81–84.

Carriere, K.C. (1994) Crossover designs for clinical trials. *Statistics in Medicine*, **13**, 1063–1069.

Farmer, E.S. and Watson, R. (1989) Promoting excellence in practice through research. In *Nursing Research in Scotland*, RCN Research Society Symposium, Edinburgh, 1 December.

Gonsalkovale, M. and Lawless, J. (1987) Looking for the perfect fit. *Nursing Times*, **83**(40), 38–39.

Grimby, A., Milson, I., Molander, U., Wiklund, I. and Ekelund, P. (1993) The influence of urinary incontinence on the quality of life of elderly women. *Age and Ageing*, **22**, 82–89.

Hall, M.R.P., MacLennan, W.J. and Lye, M.D.W. (1993) *Medical Care of the Elderly*. London: Wiley.

le Roux, A.A. (1988a) Conflict of interest. *Nursing Times*, **84**(29), 32–33.

le Roux (1988b) Firm foundations: applying the results of research based on the clinical trial design to nursing practice. In *Research Society Annual Conference*. RCN Research Society, 17 April.

McCall Smith, A. (1992) Treatment of adults with mental incapacity. In Gilhooley, M.L.M. (ed.) *Consent to Treatment*. Scottish Action on Dementia, Edinburgh, pp 7–11.

Melnick, V.L., Dubler, N.N., Weisbard, A. and Butler, R.N. (1984) Clinical research in senile dementia of the Alzheimer type: suggested guidelines addressing the ethical and legal issues. *Journal of the American Geriatrics Society*, **32**, 531–536.

Norton, C. (1987) Selecting incontinence aids. *Geriatric Nursing and Home Care*, **7**(11), 11–15.

Palmer, M.H. (1988) Incontinence: the magnitude of the problem. *Nursing Clinics of North America*, **23**(1), 139–157.

Polit, D.F. and Hungler, B.P. (1987) *Nursing Research: Principles and Methods*, third edition. Philadelphia: Lippincott.

Royal College of Physicians (1990) *Research Involving Patients*. London: RCP.

Shea, J.D. (1975) Pressure sores: classification and management. *Clinical Othopaedics and Related Research*, **112**, 89–100.

Thomas, T.M., Plymat, K.R., Blannin, J. and Meade, T.W. (1986) Prevalence of urinary incontinence. *British Medical Journal*, **281**, 1243–1245.

United Kingdom Central Council for Nursing, Midwifery and Health Visiting (1989) *Exercising Accountability: a Framework to Assist Nurses, Midwives and Health Visitors to Consider Ethical Aspects of Professional Practice*. London: UKCC.

Warren, J.W., Sobal, J., Tenney, J.H., Hoopes, J.M., Damron, D., Levenson, S., DeForge, B.R. and Muncie, H.L. (1986) Informed consent by proxy: an issue in research with elderly patients. *New England Journal of Medicine*, **315**(18), 1124–1128.

Watson, R. (1989a) Good nursing practice: the only basis for cost effectiveness. *Senior Nurse*, **9**(5), 28–29.

Watson, R. (1989b) A nursing trial of urinary sheath systems. *Journal of Advanced Nursing*, **14**, 467–470.

Watson, R. (1990) The concept of cost-effectiveness. *Nursing Standard*, **4**(31), 36–39.

Watson, R. (1992) Justifying your practice. *Nursing*, **5**(3), 13.

Watson, R. (1993) *Caring for older people*. London: Baillière Tindall.

Watson, R. (1994) Practical ethical issues related to the care of people with dementia. *Nursing Ethics*, **1**, 151–162.

Watson, R. and Kuhn, M. (1990) The influence of component parts of the performance urinary sheath systems. *Journal of Advanced Nursing*, **15**, 417–422.

2

Ethical Issues in Survey Research

Jill Rogers

The Power of the Survey

The survey is one of the most widely used methods of data gathering; it is a technique used extensively by researchers in health care, as well as by market research companies, the government and a range of other organisations. As a society we seem to have an almost compulsive need to collect information about ourselves; we collect information about our behaviour patterns, our qualifications, our voting habits, and our use of various facilities such as British Rail and hospital outpatient departments. We collect information about our attitudes to political and moral issues such as tax cuts and hanging, and on more personal topics such as our consumption of alcohol and our eating and smoking habits.

The National Health Service has a current preoccupation with collecting data through surveys, particularly to identify achievements related to the standards in the Patient's Charter. *The Hospital and Ambulance Services Comparative Performance Guide 1993–1994* (NHS, 1994), the "league table" of hospital services in England, is a good example of the ways in which data collected through surveys influence the very fabric of the health service and of professionals' and clients' perceptions of that service.

As the purchaser–provider relationship becomes embedded in the health service, there is an increasing use of surveys to identify the health care needs of local populations, to explore the acceptability of health care services, and to involve clients in many aspects of planning health care services. There are some major national surveys which underpin much health care planning. For example, the General Household Survey includes important health-related questions, and the National Birthday Trust follows the lives and health of cohorts of children born in the same week.

There are a number of ethical considerations related to survey research that are not necessarily as obvious as in studies where there is, for example, a control drug trial involving clients.

The issues discussed in this chapter have been raised by my own experience of conducting surveys within the health service. In particular, my experience has been of national surveys with groups of health service staff, predominantly practising nurses, midwives and health visitors, managers and educators. My experience of using questionnaires and interviews with these groups of staff has raised a combination of methodological and practical issues which have implications when considering the ethics of survey work.

Cartwright (1993) identified six stages of survey work involving ethical considerations: deciding whether to do a survey, sampling, the collection of the data, contents of the questionnaire, data processing, and the presentation of the results. These stages made a useful framework within which to consider my own experiences of survey work in the health services. Within this framework, I have also considered the perspectives of researchers, of participants in research and of those who use research to be able to further their practice. The RCN's guidelines *Ethics Relating to Research in Nursing* (RCN Research Advisory Group, 1993) are a valuable source of specific issues which I have attempted to relate to the framework derived from Cartwright.

I shall illustrate and discuss these six stages of survey work and related ethical considerations by drawing on three national surveys on which I was the principal researcher. These are, in chronological order:

- a survey of the career patterns of nurses, midwives and health visitors who had taken a specialist post-registration programme;
- a survey of the continuing education needs of nurses, midwives and health visitors;
- a survey of the use of distance and open learning among nurses, midwives and health visitors.

All of these surveys were funded by the Department of Health, and the results have subsequently contributed to the development of continuing professional education opportunities for practitioners.

The study of the career patterns of practitioners who had taken a post-registration study was conducted from the Joint Board of Clinical Nursing Studies, which was at the time the non-statutory body with responsibility for post-registration programmes for nurses, midwives and health visitors. The JBCNS subsequently became part of the English National Board for Nursing, Midwifery and Health Visiting. The survey was in two parts, first, a longitudinal cohort study of practitioners who had taken a post-registration programme, and second, a national survey of qualified practitioners in a sample of health districts. In both parts, questionnaires were used to collect data. The aims of the longitudinal cohort study were to provide:

- descriptive profiles of practitioners' professional and educational qualifications;
- information about why practitioners decide to take a post-registration programme in a particular speciality;
- a description of the career profiles of practitioners both before and after taking a post-registration programme;
- information about practitioners' perceptions of the usefulness of the programme to their role expectations and the demands of their subsequent jobs;
- information about practitioners' career motivations and aspirations.

The second part of the study was intended to provide a comparison group against which to compare the findings from the cohort study. The aims of the national survey of qualified nurses were to provide (Rogers, 1983):

- descriptive profiles of practitioners' professional and educational qualifications;
- descriptions of career profiles of practitioners;
- information about practitioners' career motivations and aspirations.

This study was based at the JBCNS, London. In this chapter, this study will be referred to as the career patterns study.

The second study that I shall draw on was a national survey of continuing professional education for qualified nurses, midwives and health visitors. The aim of the study was to review the provision for continuing professional education for qualified practitioners and to explore practitioners' perceptions of continuing education. The study was designed in two parts. The first part was a survey of the opportunities for continuing professional education in health authorities and in institutions of higher and further education. The second part was an in-depth study, in two district health authorities in England and Wales, of the attitudes of qualified practitioners towards continuing professional education. In the first part of the study, questionnaires were used, while in the second part, semi-structured interviews were the main data collection method (Rogers and Lawrence, 1987). This study was based at the Institute of Education, University of London. It will be referred to as the continuing education survey.

The third study was a survey of the use of distance learning materials for continuing professional education for qualified nurses, midwives and health visitors in England and Wales. The data for this study were collected through a questionnaire in a sample of district health authorities; by in-depth fieldwork in five representative district health authorities in England and Wales; and by semi-structured interviews with a sample of 275 qualified practitioners who had used distance learning materials, and semi-structured interviews with 26 education staff and 38 service-based managers in the five districts (Rogers *et al.*, 1989). This study was also based at the Institute of Education, University of London. This survey will be referred to as the distance learning survey.

Ethical Issues at Six Stages of Survey Research

1. Deciding to do the survey

The first stage at which the researcher faces an ethical consideration has to be whether the "knowledge that is being sought is not already available" (RCN Research Advisory Group, 1993). Researchers must be totally satisfied, before starting on a survey, that the information to be collected is going to contribute to the body of knowledge about the subject. A survey, particularly a national survey, inevitably involves a great many people in planning, setting up the study, agreeing the research protocols, providing data, data collection and analysis and, finally, reporting on the study. In ensuring that the information is not already available, the researcher is recognising the need not to abuse the trust of others nor to impose on them unnecessarily. As the RCN observe, "Research often requires respondents to offer their time, energy or other resources. If research makes great demands on the time and skills of nurses providing care when these are scarce resources, this may consequently be a cause of injustice to both nurses and patients" (p. 8).

In the case of each of the three studies that I was involved with, the information did not exist. The first study, the career patterns survey, was initiated, in broad outline, by the Department of Health. As I worked on the detailed project specification, it became clear that there was little or no information about the career patterns of this particular group of practitioners, although there was information about some other groups' career patterns, for example, nurses who had taken degree programmes. It was therefore possible to draw on some of the methodology from this study and to pursue some similar issues.

The second and third studies arose logically from the first. The second, the continuing education survey, was identified because of the dearth of information available about the opportunities for continuing professional education. At the time of the survey, each district health authority provided educational opportunities for nursing, midwifery and health visiting staff as part of their in-service provision. In the mid-1980s there was no overall picture of continuing education for the great majority of practitioners who were clinically based. At the same time it was known from anecdotal evidence that some practitioners were undertaking the same continuing education programme more than once for different employers. There was a clear need to build up coordinated national information so that future provision could be planned from a basis of understanding.

The third study, the distance learning survey, had a similar rationale. There was increasing use of distance learning materials within the professions and no information about the extent of this use, nor any systematic insight into the perceptions of practitioners about the use of these materials. There was research among other audiences, and a certain amount of this was relevant to our study.

Cartwright (1983) has pointed out that researchers also have to be sensitive to the possibility that they might be asked to conduct a survey in order to reduce pressure for action or to postpone uncomfortable decisions. As she says, "Determining whether or not a survey can answer the questions it is intended to is largely a technical issue: but deciding to undertake a survey when it cannot do so seems to me to be unethical if the researcher realises this, incompetent if he or she does not."

2. Sampling

The purpose of survey work, whether at local or national level, is to provide reliable findings from which generalisations can be made to the wider population. It is therefore fundamental to an effective survey that great attention is paid to the sample from whom data are collected. In health care, survey work often focuses on users of the service or on professionals working within the service. Certain public records, such as electoral registers or local tax listings can be used with no ethical problems. However, many survey researchers need to access specific groups of professionals, users or other clearly identified groups. For example, a study might wish to focus on disabled people's perceptions of the health service. An immediate ethical issue arises around how to obtain information about the identity of disabled people from medical or other records.

In my own studies, I have been concerned to access professionals at different stages of their careers. This may appear to be straightforward but there are a number of ethical issues that needed to be considered. In relation to the career patterns survey, the concern was to identify a sample of nurses, to make contact with them and invite them to participate in the study.

At the time of the study, the General Nursing Council (GNC) was the registering body, access to names and addresses of individuals was limited and practitioners were not obliged to inform the GNC of subsequent moves or changes of address. The Joint Board of Clinical Nursing Studies did not keep a listing of the addresses of practitioners who had completed programmes and there was no need for a system to trace subsequent address changes. The only possible route to identifying practitioners was through the course centres where they had taken their courses.

It was decided to write to course centres requesting the last known address of practitioners who had successfully completed programmes. A 100% response was obtained to this request. One of the issues that I am sure effected this response rate was that the research team were based at the JBCNS which was the national body responsible for approving course centres. All correspondence was sent out on JBCNS headed paper and all course centres had on-going relationships with JBCNS officers. There was therefore a certain, unspoken pressure on course centres to respond positively to our request. Being aware of this, we were particularly careful, when writing to practitioners, to explain the nature and purpose of the study, how and why they were selected and invited to take part in the study, what would be required of them and who was funding the study (RCN Research Advisory Group, 1993). We made it clear that each individual had the option to decline to participate in the study.

In the survey of qualified practitioners which was conducted in parallel with this study, we decided to draw a systematic sample of 20 health districts in England and Wales. Our intention had been to draw a sample of nurses in each district, but it became clear that there were ethical issues concerned with this plan. Districts did not necessarily have up-to-date staffing lists from which to draw a sample, and some districts were conscious of their responsibilities to their staff and did not feel able to release names even where listings existed. We therefore decided to ask each of the districts to help in distributing a brief questionnaire and explanatory letter to all practitioners employed in the selected districts. In this way, the districts did not have to provide us with any identifying information about their employees and individual practitioners could decide whether to participate in the study. The letter stressed that completion of the questionnaire was voluntary and assured complete confidentiality and anonymity. To emphasise the anonymity and to demonstrate that completed questionnaires would not be seen by their employers, we provided a freepost service so that completed questionnaires could be mailed direct to the research team.

In the continuing education survey (1987), the second part was an in-depth interview study of the attitudes of practitioners, managers and educators. A sample of health districts was selected, based on the national survey. We then needed to identify individuals in order to approach them to invite them to participate in the study.

From our previous experience we thought that districts might be reluctant to disclose details of staff. Because we were to conduct interviews, we needed to identify a smaller number of practitioners with particular characteristics. A widely distributed questionnaire would not have met our needs. We therefore adopted a different approach: we defined the criteria for selection to reflect the clinical emphasis of each district to include grade, degree of experience of continuing professional education, length of time in post, and clinical speciality. Districts were then asked to identify a certain number of practitioners to meet these criteria. This involved districts in a considerable

amount of work particularly because they did not all hold accessible informa
tion about practitioners' experience of continuing education. The study was
funded by the Department of Health, and districts were immensely helpful
in providing information for no cost to the research project. Although this
strategy involved districts in a lot of work, this approach did protect effectively the identity of individuals until the point when they were invited to
participate in the study.

While it may appear that information about participation in continuing
education activities is unlikely to raise ethical issues, it is important to remember that what is considered confidential varies from person to person and over
time. It is the responsibility of the researcher to be acutely aware of potential
ethical concerns, even where these may not appear at first sight to exist, and
to consider ways of dealing with them.

3. Collection of data

I have already touched on some of the issues concerning the collection of data
when discussing the reason for the studies, their aims and what would be
required of potential participants. There are a number of additional ethical
issues relating to the collection of data which are important to consider.

Participants in a survey must know how the information is to be used. For
example, in the distance learning survey and continuing education survey,
there was a possibility that some practitioners might be concerned that their
comments about access to distance learning and continuing education opportunities could be disclosed to their managers. This concern could have
inhibited their responses. We therefore arranged for postal questionnaires to
be returned direct to the research team using a freepost address so that
completed questionnaires were not collected within the participants' em-
ploying organisations. At the interview stage participants were assured in
writing of complete confidentiality. In survey work involving service users,
it is equally important to be sure that they fully understand the uses to which
the data will be put; users may have concerns that their treatment may be
affected by their responses, or indeed their willingness to participate in a
survey.

Related to this are the issues of confidentiality and anonymity. Researchers
should consider carefully whether they need to have contact details of
respondents. In the first of my studies of the career patterns of practitioners,
we needed to have names and addresses for participants because they were
part of a cohort study, and we planned to send them three questionnaires over
a period of time in order to track their career patterns. We made clear in our
correspondence with participants why we needed their names and addresses,
and assured them that their responses would be confidential to the research
team and that no individuals would be identified in any report of the study.

Many surveys, however, consist of a single questionnaire or interview. If this is the case, a sequential code number can be used for each respondent. For example, the aim of my survey of nurses, midwives and health visitors was to find out how much continuing professional education had been experienced by nurses in different grades, and with different lengths of service. The names of individuals were of no importance at all, provided I had information about the grade and length of service of respondents. The questionnaires were distributed by the health authority to all qualified nurses, and a reminder letter was phrased so that anyone who had already responded was thanked, while those who had not were reminded to return their question-naire. As the analysis was designed to examine differences between respondents from different grades and specialities and with differing experience, at no stage was it necessary to know the names of respondents.

Confidentiality does not necessarily mean anonymity. What is important in observing confidentiality is that an individual's responses cannot be attributed to that individual. This is an important element in the analysis and presentation of the data.

In my particular experience, because we have been interviewing professional staff and have not been concerned with clients or users of the service, ethics committee approval has been relatively straightforward. In each case a copy of the research aims and methodology was submitted together with an indication of how the work was to be reported. Each study had the support of a steering group who were responsible for advising on the on-going conduct of the survey. The participation of the steering group no doubt helped ethics committees to feel able to approve the studies.

Cartwright and Seale (1990) have commented on the variation in standards and criteria between ethics committees. In the context of their study, "Life before Death", they comment that the present system is particularly ill-equipped to deal with national studies covering several areas. They suggest that a national ethics committee might help or at least the situation would be improved if there was some agreement on the nature of research studies that should be reviewed by local committees.

Moodie and Marshall (1992) make a similar comment in relation to the Department of Health guidelines on local ethics committees. They observe that the Department of Health (1991) guidance on multicentre studies is ambivalent, it suggests that each local research ethics committee (LREC) is "free to arrive at its own decision when considering a proposal which is planned to take place in more than one area". At the same time the guidance says "committees should arrive at a voluntary arrangement under which one LREC is nominated to consider the issue on behalf of all of them". The Department guidance does not respond to Cartwright and Seale's comments that they had to complete a wide variety of forms, there has been no suggestion that a standardised form be prepared for use nationally.

One other important comment about LRECs relates to how the conduct of research may be monitored. Neuberger (1992) has drawn attention to this and recommends spot checks on research in progress to ensure that it is being carried out in accordance with the approval given by the ethics committee.

Working in the health service, or indeed any major organisation, it is essential to be aware of the need to inform all those who have an interest in the study that it is being conducted. In my studies, which have all been conducted in health districts, we have been careful to inform the senior professional, managerial and educational staff of the aims and overall conduct of the study. We have also informed staff associations. There has occasionally been an issue concerning the time taken by nursing staff either to complete a questionnaire or take part in an interview. This was resolved by discussions with employers and staff associations and full cooperation given. Indeed, with the survey of continuing education, staff associations were keen to see the results of the survey for their own forward planning.

Participation in surveys must, of course, be voluntary and participants must be fully aware of this. At the same time the research team want to achieve as high a response rate as possible and it is important to be aware of the tendency to encourage individuals to participate. This can be a particular issue where the research worker is a professional, and may be involved in the care or education of participants. In my work I was careful to employ interviewers who had no connection with the participants. I was also careful, when working from the JBCNS, to emphasise that our role as researchers was concerned with education and not with the JBCNS's organisation and monitoring functions.

It can be the case that participants in a survey ask the interviewer for information or help. I had this experience in both the continuing professional education survey and the distance learning survey. Participants would often ask for information about continuing education opportunities and available distance learning materials and for advice about the effect of participation in continuing education on their future career. We were careful to respond to such queries only after the interview was complete and only to do so if explicitly asked by the participant.

4. Contents of the questionnaire or interview schedule

There are two major ethical principles on which nursing is based (RCN Research Advisory Group, 1993). These two principles are those of doing good to people (beneficence) and doing them no harm (non-maleficence). In designing a questionnaire or interview schedule, it is important to be aware of the potential for doing harm to participants. As Oppenheim (1992) has stated, "The basic ethical principle governing data collection is that no harm should come to the respondents as a result of their participation in the research." The respondent should also have a right to privacy or to refuse to answer certain questions.

Researchers should be aware of the potential sensitivity of questions in a questionnaire or in an interview. Participants may be embarrassed or upset by questions which remind them of distressing or painful events. In my own work there have been occasions when enquiry about an individual's continuing education experience can be distressing because of the negative circumstances that surrounded the experience, for example, a negative response from a manager. Oppenheim (1992) stressed that the basic ethical principle governing data collection is that no harm should come to the respondent as a result of their participation in the research.

I have a particular concern about the extent to which information is collected that is relevant to the aims of the study. In survey work it is particularly easy to add "just one more question". Participants spend a considerable amount of time responding to questions and it is, in my opinion, unethical to collect information that is not used to address the aims of the study. Researchers are in a relatively privileged position and participants will usually do all they can to meet the researcher's requests for information. It is therefore the researcher's responsibility to make sure that all the time and information given by participants will be used to address the aims of the study.

Pilot work is valuable in identifying any questions that do not earn their keep. In my study of career patterns, the pilot study helped us to exclude questions about respondents' training schools, and the "job schedule" which asked for details of experience in nursing employment was restricted, as a result of the pilot work, to essential information with no details being collected about the names of employers. We also eliminated certain questions about employment details or perceptions of employment because respondents varied in their ability to remember events, and the data were therefore not reliable.

Selltiz *et al.* (1965) suggest a number of questions to ask when deciding about question content. They include: Is the question necessary? Just how will it be useful? Do respondents have the information necessary to answer the question? Will the respondents give the information that is asked for?

5. Data processing

Confidentiality is of particular concern in the data processing phase of survey work. As computers are used almost universally for data analysis, it is important to ensure that every safeguard is taken to maintain confidentiality for respondents. In 1987, the Data Protection Act made it necessary for those using a computer to process information to register with the Data Registrar.

This applies to anyone who is handling and manipulating information about named, identifiable individuals. Researchers should register with the Data Protection Bureau and will have to specify whether the information is being used for teaching, research or for any other purpose.

It is also important to make sure that any paper copies of names and addresses of respondents are kept safe. In my study of career patterns, we asked for names and addresses to be able to send practitioners subsequent questionnaires. We had to be careful to ensure that the listing of names and addresses was kept confidential. Although we did not have any information that could be regarded as highly sensitive such as disclosures about drug use or about sexual or delinquent activities, it was necessary to make certain that the listing could not be accessed by anyone other than the research team.

At the data processing stage, as at the questionnaire construction stage, it is important to have a clear view of the aims of the study. It can be very tempting to try to analyse "just one more" relationship but it must relate to the aims of the study. Otherwise valuable resources will be used on work that is not contributing to the overall aim of the work.

6. Presentation of the results

In the RCN's booklet, *Ethics Related to Research in Nursing* (RCN Research Advisory Group, 1993) it is stated that "Researchers have a responsibility to publish (or otherwise make available) the results of the research. This includes making available information about methods, research tools, all relevant data (including negative findings), any limitations of the research and the extent to which results obtained can be generalised." They go further and state "Researchers should take every available opportunity to disseminate and promote appropriate use of their research and should not ignore any apparent misuse."

In my own work I have been committed to disseminating the results of the research through published reports, articles and presentations at conferences and study days. With a colleague who had conducted a separate but complementary study, I organised a conference to focus on the findings from our studies, both of which were in the field of continuing professional education. The aim of the conference was to explore the implications of the two pieces of research for education and practice.

The recently published *Strategy for Research in Nursing, Midwifery and Health Visiting* stresses that "the responsibilities of the commissioners of research include the need to establish a strategic approach to dissemination" (Department of Health, 1993).

In the process of presenting the results of survey research, researchers have to be aware of the need to maintain respondents' confidentiality, regardless of whether those are individuals or organisations. When working in health authorities, it is often important for the user of the findings to have an understanding of the context of the authorities from which the data were collected. In our survey of distance learning, we conducted in-depth interviews in five health authorities. The health authorities did not wish to be named but were agreeable to our publishing a brief description of each authority. For example, we described one district in the following way:

> District Midland is set in the north-east part of the Midlands and is dominated by traditional industries, including mining. The total population of 288,000 is serviced by a total of 1885 qualified nurses of all grades and duty. The district health authority is widespread, taking in large and small rural communities, one small urban community with its own general hospital, as well as one major urban area which hosts the district general hospital. The district recently restarted its first level nurse education programme and the first of the new cohort are approaching the end of their training. The post-basic education department is situated within the Nurse Education Department; continuing professional education for midwives is organised separately by the Midwifery Unit/Education Department. The district offers a full range of clinical specialties.

Arguably this pen picture of an authority could enable the diligent reader to identify the authority. However, for the great majority of readers the identity of the authority has been concealed. The wording of this description was agreed with the authority and only used with their approval.

In the study of career patterns, the decision was taken not to identify the course centres where practitioners had completed their course. The focus of the study was the career patterns of practitioners and the extent to which they worked in the speciality of their course. There was no reason to know where they had completed the course, particularly as every course centre was approved by the Joint Board of Clinical Nursing Studies and consequently met national criteria.

There is an overarching ethical concern in relation to the presentation of research results which relates to suppression of information. It seems to me that, in general, if respondents have given their time, the research team have worked on the data and the funding organisation have monitored the research throughout, the results should be published and not suppressed. However, this is not a black and white situation, and the researcher should consider carefully whether any harm may be done by publishing any part of the results.

Becker (1978) quotes Fichter and Kolb (1953) who have presented a systematic consideration of ethical problems in reporting. They suggest that several conditions affect the problem of reporting. First, the researcher may have multiple loyalties: to those who have allowed or sponsored the study, to the source from which research funds have been obtained, to the publisher of the research report, to other researchers, to the society itself and to the community or group studied and its individual members. Second, the group under study may or may not be in a position to be affected by the published report. A historical study which describes aspects of people who will never have access to the research report poses few problems. On the other hand, a description of a contemporary community or institution can pose many problems. Third, problems can arise when the report analyses behaviour related to traditional and sacred values such as sex or religion, and also when the report deals with private rather than with public facts. Fourth, when data are presented in a statistical form, the problem of identifying an individual does not arise as it does when the mode of analysis is more anthropological.

As Becker points out, the results of survey research can cause trouble when they reveal attitudes or patterns of behaviour that some would rather not know about. Any kind of research can expose a disparity between reality and some rule or ideal, and so cause trouble. While researchers should strive for the freest possible conditions of reporting, they should also listen to their own conscience. It is not necessary to publish conclusions which do not relate to the main argument or which cause suffering out of proportion to the scientific gain of making them public.

Conclusion

Ethical concerns are evident in every aspect of nursing research, and survey research is no exception. It is clear from this analysis of the national surveys that I and colleagues have conducted that there are important concerns to be addressed by researchers who choose to use the survey method.

References

Becker, H. (1978) *Problems in the publication of field studies*. In Bynner, J. and Stribley, K.M. (eds) *Social Research: Principles and Procedures*. London: Longman Group.

Cartwright, A. (1983) *Health Surveys in Practice and in Potential, a Critical Review of Their Scope and Methods*. London: King Edward's Hospital Fund for London.

Cartwright, A. and Seale, C. (1990) *The Natural History of a Survey*. London: King Edward's Hospital Fund for London.

Department of Health (1991) *Local Research Ethics Committees*. London: Department of Health (HSG(91)5).

Department of Health (1993) *Taskforce on the Strategy for Research in Nursing, Midwifery and Health Visiting*. Leeds: Department of Health.

Fichter, J.H. and Kolb, W.L. (1953) Ethical limitations on sociological reporting. *American Sociological Review*, **18**, 96–97.

Moodie, P.C.E. and Marshall, T. (1992) Guidelines for local research ethics committees, *British Medical Journal*, **304** (16 May), 1293–1295.

Neuberger, J. (1992) *Ethics and Health Care: the Role of Research Ethics Committees in the United Kingdom*. London: King's Fund Institute.

NHS (1994) *The Patient's Charter, Hospital and Ambulance Services Comparative Performance Guide 1993–1994*. NHS Executive: Department of Health.

Oppenheim, A.N. (1992) *Questionnaire Design and Attitude Measurement*, new edition. London: Pinter Publishers.

RCN Research Advisory Group (1993) *Ethics Related to Research in Nursing*. London: Royal College of Nursing.

Rogers, J. (1983) *Follow up Study*, Vols 1 and 2. London: Department of Health.

Rogers, J. (1987) *Continuing Professional Education for Nurses, Midwives and Health Visitors*. Oxford: Ashdale Press with Austen Cornish Publishers.

Rogers, J., Maggs, C. and Lawrence, J. (1989) *Distance Learning Materials for Continuing Professional Education for Nurses, Midwives and Health Visitors*. London: Institute of Education, University of London.

Selltiz, C., Jahoda, M., Deutsch, M., and Cook, S.W. (1965) *Research Methods in Social Relations*. London: Methuen.

3

Ethical Dimensions of Action Research

Judith Lathlean

Introduction

Action research in its various forms is still relatively novel in nursing, and its validity and appropriateness as a "scientific" method to conduct investigations is only just being established. This chapter describes my experiences of undertaking a project which was aimed at evaluating an innovative scheme for the training of ward sisters in two hospitals, using an action research strategy (Lathlean and Farnish, 1984). It was my first attempt at using the methodology on such a large scale – the study was planned to take place over a three-year period – and for a project that was partially funded by a government institution, the Department of Health and Social Services (DHSS). Both of these factors, combined with the unusualness of the approach and its other characteristics, had a bearing on the conduct of the research, and in turn on the philosophical, ethical and political dimensions of the research.

I will raise a number of such issues and describe how these were addressed. For example, at the macro-level, there are concerns related to the choice of action research and the need to convince others of its worth. This process, which in turn is linked with political aspects, can in itself give rise to a situation where the researcher is tempted not to be entirely honest. Second, there is an inevitable tension between action and research and issues of power and equity within a research design that purports to be participatory, collaborative and emancipatory. Third, gaining consent to participate can be problematic, especially when there may be a fine dividing line between what people are expected to do as an accepted part of their jobs and the requirements of the endeavour as a research project. Other aspects are those of confidentiality and anonymity, the dissemination of the research findings and concerns surrounding the "ownership" of the research.

First, the scheme will be described briefly along with the chosen research design.

The Training Scheme and its Evaluation

In the late 1970s, the King Edward's Hospital Fund for London (King's Fund), motivated by the desire to improve the preparation of nurses as ward sisters, set up a new training scheme for newly appointed ward sisters in two hospitals. (The scheme is described in some detail in Allen, 1982, and King's Fund, 1982.) The idea was that, preferably prior to taking up post, the new ward sisters (trainees) would take part in a six-month programme. The first three months of the programme was spent on one of the two "training wards" (in one instance a female medical ward and in the other, a mixed surgical ward), engaging in both theoretical and practical activities geared to the job of a ward sister. They were facilitated throughout by the specially appointed ward sister for the training ward and a tutor (known together as the "preceptors"). During the second three months the trainee ward sisters embarked on their new jobs, but with "assignments" to complete and with support and visits from the tutor.

As the scheme was considered to be experimental, the King's Fund decided that a concurrent evaluation should be conducted by an independent academic institution. The Nursing Education Research Unit at Chelsea College was approached and they agreed to fund and mount an evaluation project. I was appointed as the Research Fellow and leader of the project. A professionally qualified (nurse) Research Associate was subsequently taken on to assist in the study, and to complement my expertise and background which was mainly in social and health care research and the behavioural sciences. Together we formed the research team.

My initial job specification had indicated that an action research approach would be preferable, though the reason for this early suggestion was unclear. However, during the first few months of planning it became evident that since we as researchers "sought not only to assess the effectiveness of the training scheme in preparing ward sisters for their roles, but also to assist in the development of a programme which would have widespread applicability" (Lathlean and Farnish, 1984, p. 31), an action research framework would fit.

Justifying the Methodology

As I describe elsewhere (Lathlean, 1994), the methodology for a piece of research is influenced by a number of factors including the research problem, questions or hypotheses, and the types of explanation, understanding and generalisability required. Some argue that "it is not so much a problem that determines the use of a particular research technique but a prior commitment to a philosophical position" (Bryman, 1984). In this respect a distinction is commonly made between a positivistic position (or a quantitative methodology) on the one hand and an interpretive tradition (or qualitative methodology) on the other. The former emphasises theory testing, rigorous measurement and an external perspective of a single tangible reality that is governed by laws, and which can be fragmented into variables, each capable of independent study. The latter emphasises theory generation and an internal perspective on multiple intangible realities which can only be studied holistically.

Action research is consistent with the second interpretive paradigm. Nevertheless, herein lay one of my earliest ethical dilemmas – that of the degree of honesty, integrity and courage shown in attempting to justify the methodology. The Unit I worked in was funded by the DHSS and the research was subject to scrutiny by the Chief Scientist and his scientific advisers. However, such people were much more familiar with the quantitative paradigm and thus, for example, could not understand why we did not appear to have a hypothesis that we were testing, why we had no control group and why we were not using statistical manipulations to generalise our findings. In some ways at this point it would have been easier to develop a hypothesis, to establish a control group and to utilise a complex statistical technique to satisfy our "assessors". However, this would have been wrong and not true to the methodology that we felt appropriate for the evaluation. In consequence, we had to spend weeks attempting to make out a case for the alternative approach in a way that was acceptable to those of a different methodological persuasion, but which did not compromise our principles.

Unfortunately, at the time, I was unaware of an article whereby the authors argued most cogently that "action research can base its legitimacy as science in philosophical traditions that are different from those which legitimate positivist science" (Susman and Evered, 1978, p. 582). Armed with such ammunition, alongside my enhanced understanding and experience of using action research for a number of projects, I am now more confident of my ground. Coupled with the increasing awareness of action research within the research community, the task of convincing others has become less problematic, though still something of a challenge. (For example, it is still not easy to get funding for action research where it is seen as developmental work.) In summary, action research could be said to be characterised by uncertainty, untidiness and an ongoing and continuous nature, qualities that make it a difficult though exciting research design to mount and sustain.

Tensions Between Action and Research

Action research can be described as a type of applied social research differing from other varieties in the immediacy of the researchers' involvement in the action process. It aims to contribute either to the solution of a problem, or to the development of a naturally occurring social setting *as well as* to the goals of social science (i.e. the development of knowledge or theory and sometimes reform). This is achieved by action, possibly of a collaborative nature, within an ethical framework that is mutually acceptable to researchers and practitioners or participants alike. (This definition expands on that offered in the seminal work of Rapoport, 1970, on action research.) One of the problems, however, is that the agendas of the practitioners and the researchers can be quite different. For example, practitioners may want to create change incrementally to improve practice and reach a goal, whereas researchers may prefer the action to be more tightly controlled to test effects and relationships.

Such issues proved to be difficult in this project. For a start, though the notion of "developing an ethical framework which was mutually acceptable" to all concerned was clearly ideal, this was far from easy to establish in practice. For example, the perceived relative power of the researchers in relation to the "researched" meant that participants were often hesitant about the extent to which they were "allowed" to set the parameters in conjunction with the researchers. Furthermore, the participants often seemed to view the action and the research as separate entities. Thus in their minds it was up to them to consider the ethical dimensions of the training scheme and its development, whereas it was the role of the researchers to worry about the "ethics" of the research. In reality, any early agreement as such was somewhat superficial and implicit rather than explicit. It was certainly never committed to paper, nor thought of as part of a "contract" between researcers and participants.

In terms of the methodology, at times the practitioners expected us to want a "controlled" research design, saying that maybe they should not make the changes they wished since this "might mess up the research". At other times, though, we became frustrated when it appeared evident from our research findings that an element of the scheme was not working well, yet there seemed to be a reluctance on the part of the practitioners to engage in remedial action. This gave rise to a second ethical dilemma – the extent to which we as researchers were prepared to exercise any power we may have had (or been perceived to have had) over the participants to get them to take action. The example of the problematic role of ward sister preceptor was interesting here. The "research data" clearly showed that not only were many of the trainee ward sisters confused about how they should be learning from the ward sister preceptors, but also that the "personality" of one of the ward sisters was considered to militate against effective learning. This was obviously a sensitive area, and one that we as researchers, and some of the participants, may have wished to "gloss over". However, we felt under pressure to "do something about it" and in fact, largely through our research presentations, the problem was brought to light and publicly reviewed.

This proved to be a delicate and painful process for those involved and gave rise to another ethical consideration. We were, in effect, recommending changes which were not always palatable. We were tempted and at times succumbed to the strategy of hiding behind our research findings to provide the rationale for the need for change. We should perhaps have said: "This appears to be a problem for these reasons. This seems to be the solution or the possible alternatives". Instead, we sometimes put it across as the "objective" and depersonalised findings of the research which indicated a certain pathway – it was nothing to do with us!

In considering the nature of the methodology, Webb (1990), citing Rapoport and Rapoport (1976), makes a distinction between positivist and interpretive research on the one hand and action research "in the critical" mode on the other. The former have been described as "a smash and grab raid by the researcher, who rushes in, grabs the data, and leaves the respondent to clear up the mess left behind". Conversely, "it is inherent in the philosophy of action research that the researcher and researched participate in doing the research in a way that is beneficial to both" (Webb, 1990, p. 40). Carr and Kemmis (1986) take this further in promoting action research as being emancipatory for participants; that is, it is to be engaged in order to give power to people who in other forms of research are normally relatively powerless. This is a heady brew, and whilst the logic of it is clear, in reality the tensions still exist between those who are thought to be "in the know" as far as the research is concerned and those whose business it is to take action – the practitioners. Furthermore, not all action researchers agree that they are using such a strategy to give powerless people more clout. Certainly in our project we were much more concerned with its use as a more general research approach whereby we as researchers, together with our professional colleagues were taking action in an innovative situation, and then attempting to investigate the effects of our joint actions through the use of a whole range of standard data collection methods such as observation, interviews, questionnaires and even measurement tests.

At this point the issue of collaboration within action research is pertinent. Some (e.g. Carr and Kemmis, 1986; Cohen and Manion, 1989) argue that action research is always collaborative in nature. In effect, this breaks down the distinction between researcher and researched, as suggested above by Webb (1990). Nevertheless, true collaboration raises all kinds of questions, many of which were relevant for us. For example, with whom were we collaborating and what effect did this have on decisions about all aspects of the research – the design, the data collection and the changes? Such questions proved to be a tension throughout. We felt that we could not easily "collaborate" in one sense with the trainees. We could attempt to understand the experience of the training programme from their perspective, but not involve them as such in deciding upon the research design, or how the findings were to be implemented. In any case, a new set was present during each six months. We also thought that it would be inappropriate to "collaborate" with the funders of the project – the DHSS – although we did work closely with the King's Fund, who supported the evaluation and the training scheme itself. Thus, the main people with whom we tried to develop a collaborative relationship were the preceptors. However, even this was problematic at times, especially when individuals were more used to a distant relationship between researcher and researched, in order to maintain "objectivity" as they saw it. I was bothered by this, but took comfort in the work of Powley (1976), where he suggests that in evaluating programmes, action research requires the researcher to "abandon any attempt at objectivity and declare a vested interest in the programme".

Another related aspect gave rise to concerns for us. This was to do with the interactive nature of the research design and the position of privilege that participants consider the researchers to be in. There were many times when, in the minds of the participants, things were not going quite as they had planned. Thus, we were approached on more than one occasion by frustrated "actors", pleading with us to use our authority as they saw it to "bend the ear" of the managers. For example, the dynamics amongst the trainee ward sisters in one of the institutions were problematic at one point, and the preceptors considered that one of the main reasons was a poor appointment of one trainee sister to a post. However, the preceptors felt uneasy about the prospect of raising this themselves with the implied criticism this would entail of senior managers in making the choice. So they appealed to us to intervene and to portray the "problem" as part of our research findings. We were tempted, since as colleagues we could understand their feelings, and we needed their cooperation in continuing with the project. Nevertheless, this and other occasions required some careful thought as to how far we could legitimately go to support their case.

Participation within Action Research

Gaining consent to participate within any research design is clearly important, and of course action research is no exception. However, there were a number of considerations that made it quite difficult to ensure consent to participate all of the time. Initially, all those specifically appointed to take part in the scheme were aware that the project was to be evaluated, and it could be argued that their agreement to take up their post signified consent. Likewise, the trainees also knew that they were part of an ongoing evaluation and, at least in theory, they were deemed to consent by their very participation in the programme. Nevertheless, since all newly appointed ward sisters in the institutions (and some senior staff nurses) were automatically included in the programme, was there truly an element of choice? It was certainly the case that no one was forced to complete a questionnaire or take part in an interview, but observation was used as a method throughout and it would have been virtually impossible for people to actually opt out.

The pressure for participants to cooperate was great since they knew this to be an innovative scheme with considerable vested interest on the part of the promoters for it to be successful. Also, the fieldwork (data collection) was extensive and continuous which again put pressure on all to cooperate over quite long periods of time, and within situations that were sometimes sensitive, for example, when aspects of the scheme were not considered to be working well. Indeed, this facet – the real gaining of consent to participate – was a feature that concerned me a great deal. Nevertheless, I am not sure that we found a satisfactory answer, apart from checking out at various stages whether participants were happy not only to continue to provide data, but also to have data in relation to them released more publicly and be prepared to change where felt necessary.

Confidentiality and Anonymity

Being able to guarantee both confidentiality and anonymity was not only very problematic but at times inappropriate. In a research design where it is important to feed back findings to a group of participants in order for the group to reflect upon them, and make decisions about what action, if any, needs to ensue, confidentiality cannot always be maintained. Yet we were sometimes having to cope with difficult and sensitive issues. For example, an assumption was made in the plans for the scheme that only those people with a certain level of clinical competence would be appointed to posts as ward sisters. The programme was to be about the development of managerial, leadership, personnel and research skills, rather than the development of clinical skills. However, it became evident from some of our early observations in the clinical setting and interviews with preceptors who were working with the trainees that this assumption was far from correct with a minority of the trainees. Clearly, with such "findings", it would have been invidious to identify individuals, though the general point of the need to improve selection procedures was an important aspect. Thus, it required a great deal of tact on our part to present findings in such a way that individuals were not compromised, but that the real issues were exposed. This was done, for example, by presenting findings in a more "theorised" way, so that concepts (e.g. of different ways of learning from a ward sister preceptor in a practice setting) were discussed, rather than the specific examples which gave rise to the need to talk about the concept in the first place. This is obviously a concern with other designs, but where the expectation is that findings will be used to change and modify, this problem is exacerbated.

Another related concern was the phenomenon we labelled: "Who said that?" On many occasions we were attempting to present our evidence to substantiate our recommendations when it was necessary perhaps to present material that was critical of individuals or groups. We were often challenged to reveal our sources. At times it was extremely difficult to maintain confidentiality or to retain anonymity. We tried as far as we could, and when it seemed neither possible nor productive we made every effort to gain the permission of those involved to enable us to talk quite openly about the issues.

Publishing the Findings

Confidentiality and anonymity are a concern too when publishing the findings, and one that is shared with case study research. Those involved with the project made a clear decision fairly early on that the two institutions would be identified. The scheme had become well known and it would have been very artificial to attempt to make the institutions anonymous themselves when preparing documentation that would be publicly available. Within each institution, obviously some individuals were unique; for example, there were only two chief nurses, two ward sister preceptors and two tutors. It was unnecessary to name them; their identity was clear just by reference to their title. This was less so for the trainees and some other participants. For example, each six-month course in both institutions had at least two trainees, and many of the findings talked about the trainees as a much larger group. But still the worry was always there.

The only way around this seemed to be to allow all relevant participants to see all the draft versions of reports, prior to their publication. In this way they could both challenge our interpretations and ask for any sensitive aspects to be removed. This we did throughout, but since most of the early documents were only for consumption by a relatively small audience (i.e. those directly involved in the research and the funding institutions) this did not appear to cause undue concern. Nevertheless, it was with great trepidation that I sent the final draft report to all the key actors. I was concerned about anonymity; I was worried that they might become defensive and wish to disassociate themselves from it. Their reactions were surprising! Several simply did not reply by the (very generous) deadline we gave them. Others just said: "its fine". There was only one substantial reply – from one of the tutors. She made remarks on several of the parts though mainly by way of commentary rather than critique. But her one abiding overall judgement was: "I find it interesting, but a bit bland. I feel you should have been a lot harder, a lot more critical of some of the things we did or did not do! I for one consider the impression given of me to be a great deal more positive than I feel I deserve!" I concluded that in our efforts to be fair, to retain confidentiality and to be anonymous perhaps we had lost some of the essence of the experience. It was hard, difficult and problematic work at times, and maybe we had not represented it as it was, and how at least one participant considered we should.

The Ownership of the Research

One of the issues which is often considered in action research is that of the "ownership" of the research – to whom does the research "belong", both in terms of the process and the outcomes. As mentioned above, some hold the view that types of research other than action research are undertaken primarily to serve the interests of the researcher rather than the participants. It follows from this that if action research is promoted as a collaborative venture then many aspects of it must be considered as shared – for example, the data collected, the interpretations of it, and certainly the material presented. This can give rise to difficulties if, for example, the researchers are commissioned to do the research by a body that has no direct relationship with the participants: they may feel that the research should belong to them rather than collectively to those who took part in it.

To a certain extent this was a concern for us, since the DHSS clearly had an interest in the research – its design, conduct and findings – yet no involvement with the practitioners. Fortunately, though, apart from ensuring that the research was being conducted appropriately through the mechanism of the Chief Scientist's visits to the Research Unit, the DHSS did not intervene in the study; they allowed us to work with the participants in the way that we chose, and we were able to decide (along with participants) what would become public and how.

This is also a potential problem when people choose to undertake action research for a higher degree. Here, they must be able to present a thesis or dissertation that is clearly their own work, yet the extent to which it is based on a joint effort has ethically to be recognised.

Conclusion

In many ways, action research is little different from other forms of research in the kind of ethical dilemmas and considerations that are raised. However, certain features of the approach give rise to particular problems, such as the nature of the relationship between researchers and researched; the fact that action research is invariably based within one particular context and thus potentially identifiable; and the access that is often afforded to the researchers to sensitive information by the long exposure that they have within the action setting.

The action research project described in this chapter was undertaken at a time when such studies were relatively unusual, and the literature gave few guidelines. Since this project, I have been involved in other action research projects. Clearly, this accumulation of experience has helped, but nevertheless some important ethical considerations remain. Perhaps one of the most pertinent is that of the length of time that some action research studies take. Can the investment of time, resources and energy be justified unless the endeavour is going to develop and expand nursing knowledge as well as the understanding of the researchers and participants engaged in it? To this end, I am committed to the promotion of high-quality action research in nursing and health care.

References

Allen, H.O. (1982) *The Ward Sister – Role and Preparation*. London: Baillière Tindall.

Bryman, A. (1984) The debate about quantitative and qualitative research: a question of method or epistemology? *British Journal of Sociology*, **35**(1), 75–92.

Carr, W. and Kemmis, S. (1986) *Becoming Critical: Education, Knowledge and Action Research*. Lewes: The Falmer Press.

Cohen, L. and Manion, L. (1989) *Research Methods in Education*, third edition. London: Routledge.

King's Fund (1982) *Ward Sister Preparation: A Contribution to Curriculum Building*. London: King's Fund Centre.

Lathlean, J. (1994) Choosing an appropriate methodology. In Buckeldee, J. and McMahon, R. *The Research Experience in Nursing*. London: Chapman and Hall.

Lathlean, J. and Farnish, S. (1984) *The Ward Sister Training Project*. London: Nursing Education Research Unit, Chelsea College, University of London.

Powley, T. (1976) *Action research*. Unpublished paper. National Children's Bureau.

Rapoport, R.N. (1970) Three dilemmas of action research. *Human Relations* **23**(6), 499–513.

Rapoport, R. and Rapoport, R.N. (1976) *Dual Career Families Re-examined*. London: Martin Robertson.

Susman, G.I. and Evered, R.D. (1978) An assessment of the scientific merits of action research. *Administrative Science Quarterly*, **23**, 582–602.

Webb, C. (1990) Partners in research. *Nursing Times*, **86**(32), 40–44.

4

Ethnography in Clinical Situations: an Ethical Appraisal

Steven Ersser

Introduction

The term ethnography refers to an approach to qualitative research. Ethnographers work closely with those in the social scene or field under study. Planning such research requires attention to the negotiation of access to the clinical area, the identity conveyed by the researcher, the role they adopt, the relationships to be formed and the way they intend to leave the setting. These activities impinge upon those participating in the study and raise ethical issues. Prominence is given to four major areas of ethical consideration that arise from ethnographic work, as follows:

(1) avoiding or limiting deception;
(2) protecting the autonomy of the participants;
(3) avoiding or limiting intrusion/respecting the welfare of participants;
(4) encouraging ethical use of research findings.

These overlapping themes provide a framework for exploring the ethical implications of ethnographic research in clinical situations. I will draw primarily on my experience of conducting an ethnographic study of nursing in a hospital setting as an illustration.

Ethnographic research involves the description and analysis of aspects of culture. Cultural knowledge provides the framework from which people interpret their experience and organise their actions. The ethnographer is concerned with the meaning of actions and events to those people under study (Spradley, 1979).

The illustrative study examined nurses and patients' views on the therapeutic effect of nursing. It aimed to discover whether nurses and patients held views on the consequences of nurses' actions for patients and, if so, to identify the nature of these views. Four clinical settings across three provincial hospitals were selected. These included two general medical wards, a neurology and a dermatology ward. The convenience sample consisted of 17 cases, which included seven adult patients and ten nursing staff. Three data collection methods were employed; use of a self-recorded diary and ethnographic interviews (semi-structured informal style). The nurses also engaged in a group discussion. A primary question was used to trigger data collection; its format was varied slightly according to whether the information was for a nurse or a patient. Most data collection activities were conducted on the ward. The process of data collection and analysis conformed to the grounded theory approach (Glaser and Strauss, 1967). Further details are given in Ersser (1991).

Fieldwork is a central activity in any ethnographic study. It involves an observer maintaining face-to-face involvement with the members of a particular social setting for the purposes of scientific inquiry (Johnson, 1975). The terms field research and participant observation are often used interchangeably. The degrees and types of involvement in the field may vary for each study.

As field sites, hospitals have distinctive qualities that may influence the conduct and outcome of fieldwork and therefore ethical conduct. An important factor is the vulnerability of participants, both patients and staff. Such conditions have consequences for the access arrangements of the researcher and the avoidance of undue intrusion.

A reflexive approach was taken to research. This involved recognition of the researcher's integral part of the social world under study (Hammersley and Atkinson, 1983). In practice the researcher monitors their own actions in the field using a fieldwork journal. This provides a way of gaining a better understanding of the process of data collection. This helped to raise my awareness of ethical issues in the field. Journal entries are given in this chapter (indicated in the text by "FWJ", the number of the journal and the page reference). Some specific ethical issues related to ethnographic research in clinical situations are now explored.

1. Avoiding or Limiting Deception

... the fieldworker often has to be interactionally deceitful in order to survive and succeed (Punch, 1986, p. 71).

The researcher will normally be a stranger to the social situation that they are studying and therefore they will need to gain the trust of those involved. This includes consideration of how to present themselves in the field so as to balance the need to collect useful data with the need to limit deception. The fieldworker may be deceptive concerning the research purpose, the revelation of their identity, the use of research methods and by promises (Punch, 1986). Participants may feel deceived when undue ambiguity arises in the researcher's identity. This may disrupt trust in the researcher and therefore impede data collection activities.

Two particular issues are now explored further:

* relationship with the informants and role in the field;
* impression of role given to others.

Relationship with the informants and role in the field

Fieldworkers may adopt various observational roles. These roles reflect the degree to which the researcher participates in the social life of the clinical setting and has both ethical and research implications. Data collection requires the researcher to negotiate a role in the field.

The concept of participant observation is central to understanding ethnographic research conduct and its implications. It refers to a variety of activities in the fieldwork area. Conventionally, the participant observer is involved intimately in the social activities of those under study, but the degree of involvement varies. The anthropological origins of ethnography are based on the belief that to understand a society there is a need for the researcher to be immersed in it and be required to think, see, feel and sometimes act as a member of its culture (Powdermaker, 1966). Thus the opportunities for direct observation presented by participation in the primary social activities of the setting become the focus, for example, in her study of hospice care James (1984) worked as a staff nurse.

A broader interpretation of participant observation may be found in contemporary ethnographic studies in the sociological field. From a reflexive stance, any way in which researchers engage in the field may be seen as participant observation in a wider sense.

> Interviews must be viewed, then, as social events in which the interviewer (and for that matter the interviewee) is a participant observer (Hammersley and Atkinson, 1983, p. 126).

In the study illustrated here, I entered the field as a researcher and did not directly participate in nursing activity. Some field roles will involve a greater degree of participation in the conventional social roles in the field and so may heighten the risk of deception. Gold (1958) described a range of field roles which the researcher may adopt. I adopted the role of observer-as-participant role which Gold says involves "one-visit interviews" (p. 377) and involved participation in social encounters. Time was spent visiting the ward, waiting around to approach patient participants, sitting in the office where nurses would come for coffee or nursing reports. These served as useful opportunities to see nurses engaging in conversation and provided contextual information for the study. In an ethnographic study of student nurses, Melia (1987, p. 191) adopted the observer-as-participant role. Her fieldwork took place in the students' flats. Towell's (1975) study of psychiatric nursing involved him "participating as a research worker in the daily life of the organisation being studied" (p. 39).

Although the researcher's identity may not be concealed they may fail to be completely open about their motives (Bulmer, 1982). This could have applied in some cases to my observations made during informal contact with the participants. Participant observation may be covert whereby an extended period of time is spent in the study setting with the researcher concealing their role whilst pretending to play some other (Bulmer, 1982). Covert studies have been conducted in clinical settings (Caudill *et al.*, 1952; Rosehan, 1973). The desirability of covert research is subject to controversy. Douglas (1976) states that the primary objective of sociology should be to search for truth and the ends may justify the means. However, Munhall (1988, p. 151) argues that: "The therapeutic imperative of nursing (advocacy) takes precedence over the research imperative (advancing knowledge) if conflict develops." Bulmer (1982, p. 250) concludes that the case for the use of covert methods is considerably exaggerated.

Impression of role given to others

An issue directly related to the limitation of deception in the field is the role impression created by the researcher. Those participating in the study will seek to determine who will be the audience for their accounts subsequently and judge the trustworthiness of the researcher. This may have an important influence on the participant's willingness to disclose information. The difficulties of avoiding deception whilst attempting to be effective as a fieldworker are now explored.

Limiting deception

The researcher must ensure that those in the fieldwork area are not unduly deceived in the course of fieldwork. But it is often difficult to totally avoid deception in practice. I found myself presenting different identities related to my various roles outside the field. I reflected on my initial contact with the first ward and the various impressions I could create:

> I introduced myself [to a nurse] by name and as "research nurse". I did not consciously plan to give myself this title – it came to me spontaneously. I could have called myself "research student" or "researcher". . . . I wanted to convey something which would be common to myself and the staff. This made me aware of how I introduce myself. I say important because of the possible connotations

of each label or title. For example, "research nurse" clearly conveys the fact that I am a nurse and so I will have some insight into the work of the staff [and from the patients' point of view possibly an "expert"]. "Research student" may convey the "learning to do research impression", which although true is a relative statement since all researchers continue to learn about research. To use these terms [as I did in the letter of introduction to doctors and sisters] may have perhaps induced a lack of confidence . . . a particular concern when dealing with vulnerable patients. Use of the title "researcher" may convey that I have little in common with them [nurses] . . . [and] may affect my ability to develop rapport with participants. In practice I found that I would use a variety of "titles" which convey a whole set of impressions (FWJ1, pp. 6–8).

No deliberate attempt was made to deceive the informants as to my identity and role as a researcher. I introduced myself with the consistent features of trying to convey that I was a nurse and a researcher. I also had to consider how the full disclosure of my identity would affect my relationship with the participants and the data collected.

I noted in my fieldwork journal that the interpretation of my age in the field appeared to play a part since it helped me to remain covert as a tutor due to my relatively young appearance. Burgess (1984) describes how his age influenced his role in an ethnographic study of a school.

The issue of the acceptable use of deception in field research has been raised by several authors. It is said that the practice is both recognised and accepted (Bok, 1982). Punch (1986, p. 41) argues that some measure of deception is acceptable in some areas where the benefits of knowledge outweigh the harms and where the harms have been minimised by following convention on confidentiality. One suggestion made is that the researcher need not always be brutally honest, direct and explicit with one's research purpose. Similarly, Hammersley and Atkinson (1983) argue that to be explicit about the purposes and procedures of ethnographic studies is often neither possible nor desirable. Typically, research problems arise in the course of fieldwork and so the research aims are considered tentative at the outset of the study.

The studies of Liebow (1967) and James (1984) highlight the importance of personal appearance, dress and demeanour, in conveying specific identities to those in the field. James' (1984) study of hospice nursing exemplifies the subtle concerns of the ethnographer of wanting to avoid deception.

To maintain my identity as a researcher, what I wore to work became of symbolic significance. I was in a quandary, as I did not want to deliberately obscure my identity to pretend I was not doing research, but also wanted to be accepted as one of the team, though the administrators wanted me to be visibly different. The white coat was discarded in favour of a nursing dress, but I was not to have a hat or epaulettes which denote the stage and type of training (James, 1984, p. 136).

Similarly, I was conscious of my appearance and the messages it may convey in the clinical field. I wore mufti since I did not have a clinical role and was conscious of a need to achieve a balance between approachability and respectability in the eyes of patients. For most patients it appeared that I was accepted as a nurse, not only a researcher. Different types of participants and different contexts may require the researcher to adapt to maintain their social competence (Hammersley and Atkinson, 1983).

Researcher and nurse

As an observer and a nurse there were implications for the limitation of deception and intrusion in the field. The clinical setting is an alien environment for many researchers. Ethical and methodological issues are raised here, both in terms of the risk of abusing one's position as a nurse and one's effectiveness as a fieldworker. For the second stage of fieldwork (six months) I worked as a research assistant. I felt it was important that staff continued to know that I was a nurse to convey that the setting would be familiar to me and that I could engage with patients in a sensitive way. In an ethnographic study of school, Beynon (1983) describes how it was useful to present himself as a former teacher. When engaging with patients I emphasised that I was "a nurse doing research". I believe this was of great significance in terms of the patient's willingness to disclose to me throughout the study.

2. Protecting the Autonomy of the Participants

The participants of a study have a right to be informed about the nature of the research situation and the implications for themselves. Patients are of course a vulnerable group in this respect. Consent to participate in the study has to be informed and freely given. It also requires ongoing negotiation (Munhall, 1988).

Letters of invitation were written for each of the participants outlining the purpose of the research, my request for their involvement, the nature of the research activity and an explanation that they were under no obligation to participate, nor remain in the study. It was also necessary to reassure patients that their decision not to be involved would have no implications for their care.

The consent sought was of a verbal nature. At the time I felt the formality surrounding the use of a written consent form would risk generating unnecessary suspicion. However, today I feel that gaining written consent would be desirable practice. A verbal explanation of the purpose of the research was also provided at the first meeting. A follow-up visit after approximately 24 hours was intended to give the person an opportunity to consider whether they wished to participate. Subsequent visits gave other opportunities to discuss the details to be given, the aims, methods and sponsors of the study, the nature of their involvement and rights and how I wanted to use the data.

Informants were given an opportunity on each occasion we met to ask any questions or raise any concerns. I also encouraged them to discuss the issue with the ward sister who knew about the study. Consent was also sought to consult the patients' nursing notes to obtain basic background details.

A particular problem of informed consent with qualitative studies is that their nature precludes detailed prior knowledge being given to the participants about what events will occur (Cassel, 1980). For example, whilst I could gain consent for the people to participate in interviews, the number of interviews could not be specified in advance. I used the judgement of the charge nurse to guide me as to who were well enough to be invited to participate. The diary question guidelines stated that the patient was free to withdraw at any time or temporarily suspend their involvement over the five days of diary writing by notifying the ward sister.

The difficulties of ensuring that consent is freely given is exemplified by an incident in which a patient felt an obligation to participate. Ann was a frail woman in her eighties with arterial leg ulcers. She had not been suggested by the ward sister, although the nurses felt that she might be a possible participant. Ann had a poor attention span but showed a willingness to help me. I started to explain the study by first reading her a letter of introduction. She remarked she could not read the small print. Ann then explained that she had been involved in a research situation previously and this had caused her anxiety and headaches, despite her intentions to try to help the researcher. She remarked that her daughter may fear that this would happen again. It became clear here that Ann should be supported to decline involvement.

It was emphasised to all potential participants that I was studying an aspect of nursing care which would not involve my making judgements about the performance of the nurses involved. This was reinforced by the ward sister who knew a little more about the study. Despite the efforts to ensure informed consent, I observed that there were limits as to what potential participants, especially patients, wanted to know about the study.

3. Avoiding or Limiting Intrusion/Respecting the Welfare of Participants

Research into social life is intrusive by nature. There is therefore a need to protect the welfare of participants, especially the sick. To enhance the validity of their studies, ethnographers attempt to get "close" to those under study, to understand those aspects of their social life which are often not directly disclosed. This refers to the participants' cultural knowledge rather than their intimate personal details. Intrusion can be seen in terms of being an observer in areas which would otherwise be private, which may be problematic in sensitive settings such as hospitals.

Two major features of ethnographic fieldwork pose a risk of unwanted and unnecessary intrusion; preparation for access and negotiating entry into the field and the nature of ethnographic research.

Preparation for access and negotiating entry into the field

Negotiating access is a balancing act (Hammersley and Atkinson, 1983, p. 72).

The way in which the researcher is permitted to gain entry has ethical implications and may reveal analytical ideas about the organisation itself. Researchers may be seen as critics or experts (Hammersley and Atkinson, 1983). There is the need to consider who should give the researcher permission to approach hospital patients and staff and how this should be regulated. Those who exercise control over access to the setting and information are termed "gatekeepers" (Burgess, 1984).

My ability to gain access was influenced by my role in the field and the familiarity with the setting as a nurse in my own culture and this fact probably significantly influenced my ability to negotiate access at varying levels. This credibility advantage for some nurse researchers has been highlighted (Olesen and Whittaker, 1967). As a nurse, I was equipped to respond sensitively to the contingencies of the hospital setting and the practicalities of fieldwork, to minimise intrusion to the patient and avoid harm during fieldwork. For example, I was independent in helping patients to move to interview areas for privacy such as "Nina", who had a parenteral feeding pump, catheter and wound drain and could not walk unaided.

The gatekeepers included the local district research ethical committee, Directors of Nursing Service (DNS) for each hospital, the medical consultants on the wards from whom the patient informants would be invited to participate, the charge nurse for each ward area and the potential and actual informants. A check-list was used in the field as a prompt for the main access and sampling procedures.

The district research ethics committee required most research studies to be submitted for ethical approval. Approval was sought prior to each fieldwork stage. Once approval was obtained the letter of acceptance was made available at each stage of negotiating access. An appointment was then made to meet each of the three Directors of Nursing after a letter of introduction had been sent. Careful consideration was needed as to whom it would be appropriate to contact first within the organisation. I risked breaking the trust of those within the organisation should I not negotiate access appropriately.

> . . . although it was thought to be correct protocol to approach the DNS first, I had considered whether an informal brief introductory contact with the sisters on the proposed study wards would be better. This may offset any alienation that may arise from ward sisters who felt that in some way the research was

being imposed upon them. In practice I felt confident that the accepted protocol was the best approach. Not only because it was possible that approaching ward sisters before gaining permission for access could alienate me from the DNS – the key gatekeepers. Also I felt sufficiently confident that should I approach a sister who was unhappy to involve her ward in the research, then I would happily withdraw because of the level of cooperation involved in the design (SWJ1, p. 5).

No problems emerged from this approach. The letter was followed up by a telephone call to seek feedback and clarify issues prior to meeting. Knowing two of the three Directors helped to ease my access at this stage considerably. One DNS wanted to give details of the study at the next senior nurses' meeting of the hospital to seek their reaction. I was conscious of Atkinson's (1981) study of the education of medical students and Dingwall's (1980) study of health visitor training which highlighted how the powerful within an organisation may control access to those in a subordinate position.

The ward sisters were contacted by a letter of introduction and a telephone call where I made a request to meet. All gave their full support to the study, but the risk of intrusion was illustrated by one episode in a general medical ward. The first problem was that my arrival coincided with the ward report and, more importantly, arriving in a situation in which the ward sister was under considerable stress. It only emerged subsequently that beds were being closed on the ward and the sister was due to leave the ward within the month, after being in post for seven years. The issue of bed closure made it easier to offer my withdrawal from the ward prior to data collection so as to minimise any feelings of awkwardness for the ward sister.

Relations with the gatekeepers

Ethical conduct in the field depended on the relationships I formed with gatekeepers and those in the field and therefore the promotion of trust. The relations I developed with the gatekeepers had ethical implications. The ward sisters played a significant role as sponsors by helping with access through conveying their trust in me and helping me prepare for fieldwork. Together with a courtesy letter, the doctors often relied upon the nurses' acceptance of the study from the remarks of the ward sisters, and so they acted as crucial gatekeepers. The classic ethnographies of street gangs by Whyte (1981) and Liebow (1967) are examples of the value of the researcher having a sponsor in the field who can help them to gain access. Being a nurse and having worked in two of the three hospitals involved in the study gave me advantages in securing a favourable working relationship quickly. But due care was needed to ensure that the ward sisters felt able to act in such a way as to respond to any concerns or doubts of their patients and staff who did not want to participate.

Some practical difficulties emerged in recruiting participants which illustrate the risk of intrusion for patients. A few expressed fears about the purposes of the study. For example, one patient seemed to think that I might have been a "management" spy:

> Tracey turned off the t.v. She was an experienced patient, having to be admitted about three times a year for treatment of psoriasis . . . Introduced myself as "SE, a researcher at the . . ." I explained that I was here to conduct a research study in which I would like her to participate, but which she was under no "pressure" to consent to. . . . Tracey's response became a little guarded. Reluctance was evident. She said she was always "suspicious of this sort of research" (FWJ3, p. 6).

I made it clear to Tracey that the study was my own and not sponsored by anyone else but decided that, with her strong feelings of mistrust, I would not pursue her recruitment any further. With hindsight, my introduction here may have not placed sufficient emphasis on the fact that I was a nurse and I could have made more explicit the purpose and audience for the research.

Preventing the exploitation of the informants

The foregoing also indicates the difficulty for the researcher in achieving the fine balance between their attempts to build trust whilst avoiding undue intrusion. Beynon (1983) highlights the risk of researchers being exploitative in the field by being friendly in return for data. As a nurse I had a genuine interest in the welfare of patients and my colleagues and took opportunities to demonstrate this. Usefully, certain fieldwork activities helped to reinforce this position. For example, the ethnographic interview gave opportunities for normal conversation through the use of descriptive questions early in the interview ("What brought you into hospital?" "What has it been like working on this ward?"). These helped to build trust as well as providing theoretical insights.

It is not inevitable that all aspects of the research endeavour will be experienced negatively by those in the field. For example, the pace of ward life often made it difficult for nurses to have a prolonged conversation with patients. Most participants therefore responded positively to the conversational features and informal style of the ethnographic interview. These interviews also assisted my access and the development of rapport since many patients found the interviews satisfying and as providing a valuable opportunity to express themselves. Wax (1971) referred to the tendency of informants to talk freely because they want someone to talk to. This is illustrated by Nina, an elderly woman who had been in hospital for quite a while and was lonely because she could not walk.

> When I arrived various things had happened to Nina; her ileostomy drainage tube become detached and leaked over her clothes and she also needed to go to the toilet. I checked whether or not she felt up to the interview, she said

"yes" . . . Nina was quite keen to continue. I think it was clear that she enjoyed our "chats" together (as she saw them). In many ways we had become "friends". I too enjoyed seeing Nina; I felt we had developed good rapport. We got on together very well. I felt our "conversation" just occurred very naturally. I had to consciously think "I had better get started" (FWJ2, pp. 70–71).

I called a nurse to help Nina. Although a nurse, it was inappropriate for me as a researcher to assist her in such sensitive circumstances.

When reflecting on the diary question in the nurses' group discussion, several expressed guilt due to the disparity between what they felt they ought to do and what they could achieve in practice. I had to reinforce that I was trying to understand how they viewed the effects of their work as it was and not how it ought to be. However, some nurses welcomed the opportunity for them to "tell it as it is" and appeared to benefit from the research activity. The keeping of a diary about their work and having an opportunity to discuss it through the interview was valued by several nurses. Several described the value of their reflections on the effect of their actions on the patient. One nurse asked me to join her for a drink after her interview and went on to explain how her involvement had helped her to understand the basis for her dissatisfaction with her work.

The nature of ethnographic research

Ethnographic research involves making public the things said and done in private (Hammersley, 1990). This threat to privacy can be experienced as intrusive by those in the field. The informal character of the interview situation could enable sensitive information to emerge. For example, one patient "Laura" expressed problems with aspects of her care concerning the staff's sensitivity to her as a patient with an existing disability. I encouraged her to put her views to those staff she could trust. "Laura" said she had felt a little exposed sharing information honestly in the diary (FWJ1, p. 35). I acknowledged that I understood how she must have felt and how I valued her trust in me but attempted to reassure her of confidentiality and her right not to disclose information should she not want to.

Being a researcher with nursing background had disadvantages. By revealing my identity as a nurse, I was at risk of allowing patients to develop inappropriate expectations of me as a nurse. There was also a risk of creating momentary blurring of my role as a researcher and that of a nurse. Robinson and Thorne (1988) argue that the public are unlikely to be aware of the subtle distinctions between clinical and research roles. Thus their consent may be based on the expectations of the researcher as a nurse. Like Finch (1986) I was surprised by the readiness of the participants to disclose to me. I also frequently reflected on my concern about making excessive intellectual demands on the informants. A crucial balance had to be achieved between pursuing meaning in the interview and not unduly disrupting the "ordinary" quality of exchange.

Protecting confidentiality and anonymity

Attempts to limit intrusion and maintain privacy were also made by protecting confidentiality and anonymity. Assurances were given to all informants that all data would remain anonymous and confidential, but I sought their permission to use a limited amount of anonymous printed data. This was described as a copy of the diary and some excerpts from an interview written out, for teaching and publication purposes. All informants agreed to this.

Each participant was identified by a colour-coded sticker on tapes and transcripts. All transcripts were preceded by a single code letter in place of names. In the fieldwork journal pseudonyms were used. All data tapes were kept in a locked filing cabinet accessible only to the researcher. It was important to make clear to all informants that whilst I was working closely with the ward sister, she would not be party to any information given to me by them. The secretarial staff assisting me with transcription were told of their responsibilities in protecting the confidentiality of the data.

The National Institute for Nursing (1993) *Code of Conduct for Researchers* was developed after the study was complete. Here, it is suggested that the researcher considers the difficult issue of who has ownership of the information and whether the data provider has a right to ask for confidential information to be destroyed. This issue was not discussed with the informants.

4. Ethical Considerations in the Use of Ethnographic Research Findings

The ethical considerations surrounding ethnographic research apply also to the use of the findings in practice. These include protecting confidentiality and anonymity on publication, the responsibility of offering informants a chance to hear about the findings of the study and the appropriate use of ethnographic research findings.

Confidentiality and anonymity within publications

Hammersley (1992) describes how the ethnographer is in a position to exercise power over those being studied in the course of publishing their work. Despite careful attempts to protect the anonymity and confidentiality of the study participants and the study setting, there can be difficulties in maintaining these on publication. Burgess (1984) says the researcher has to make decisions about what to include, exclude, disguise and make public. Although the use of pseudonyms is said to be common in field studies, he says it often remains possible to identify individuals, institutions and locations. Care was needed in my study to avoid any indications that may lead readers to make assumptions about locations which I may independently frequent and which relate to my professional (non-research) work.

Feeding back the findings to the study participants

Thought must be given to providing opportunities to inform participants about the study findings. Those working in public service organisations are likely to want to know what insights have been gained in the course of the study. There is also a professional requirement to communicate research findings to nursing colleagues. Several opportunities were created in this study to convey intermediate findings to the informants. Nurses and patients showing keen interest were offered a brief report on the completion of the study. Problems were found locating nurses undergoing frequent job changes. I also gave several advertised open talks on the study across the health authority and at some national conferences. The location for the fieldwork remained strictly anonymous.

Appropriate use of ethnographic research findings

Ethnographers, particularly when working in applied fields such as nursing, have a responsibility to help policy makers understand the nature of ethnographic research, its value and applicability, as well as it limitations. Caution is needed among policy makers and clinical staff who use qualitative research findings. They are more likely to be familiar with studies such as surveys or experiments, in which emphasis is placed on the scope for generalising the findings to other situations. Researchers need to help those reading their studies to gain understanding of the focus with qualitative studies. This includes the in-depth description and analysis of particular situations and cases, with an emphasis on the interpretations made of those under study. The appropriate use of such has received little attention in the nursing literature. The representative features of all types of research study is important. However, the sampling methods used in qualitative studies, often involving a relatively small number of cases, requires that care is taken in attempting to extrapolate from the cases. Careful review and interpretation of the study and its findings are required. The approach is not statistical in nature as with quantitative studies, but instead it relies on the ability of the user to carefully review the specific features of the setting and the cases involved and to identify areas of similarity or difference (theoretical inference) (Clyde-Mitchell, 1983). Hammersley (1992, p. 6) highlights the need for caution in attempting to use ethnographic findings to provide solutions to immediate practical problems.

Conclusions

Conducting an ethnographic study within a sensitive field such as a hospital with its various vulnerable groups necessitates that great care is taken to anticipate and review the adverse consequences of the researcher's actions. The relatively close social involvement with those engaged in the study serves to heighten the ethical challenges facing the ethnographic researcher. Hammersley (1992) argues that such research is not intrinsically exploitative. He reminds us that the power of the researcher over the practitioner is limited due to the researcher's weak position in having to request and negotiate access. But, once access to the organisation has been obtained, there is the risk of intrusion in the course of data collection. The ethnographer, who also has experience as a nurse, is both advantaged and disadvantaged. Greater opportunities may be available due to one's familiarity with the clinical field, although there is a risk of ethical blind spots existing when the roles of nurse and researcher are blurred. Nurses conducting field research need to give adequate attention to openly reporting the ethical dimensions of their work and to informing others of where lessons have been learnt.

References

Atkinson, P. (1981) *The Clinical Experience*. Farnborough: Gower.

Beynon, J. (1983) Ways-in and staying-in: fieldwork as problem solving. In Hammersley, M. (ed.) *The Ethnography of Schooling: Methodological Issues*. Diffield: Nafferton.

Bok, S. (1982) Freedom and risk. In Bulmer, M. (ed.) *Social Research Ethics*. New York: Holmes & Meier.

Bulmer, M. (ed.) (1982) *Social Research Ethics*. London: Macmillan.

Burgess, R. (1984) *In the Field*. London: George Allen & Unwin.

Cassel, J. (1980) Ethical principles for conducting fieldwork. *American Anthropologist*, **82**, 28–41.

Caudill, W., Redlich, H., Gilmore, and H. Brody, E. (1952) Social structure and interaction processes on a psychiatric ward. *American Journal of Orthopsychiatry*. **22**, 314–334.

Clyde-Mitchell, J. (1983) Case and situation analysis. *The Sociological Review*, **31**(2), 187–211.

Dingwall, R. (1980) Ethics and ethnography. *Sociological Review*, **28**(4), 871–891.

Douglas, J.D. (1976) *Investigative Social Research*. Beverly Hills: Sage.

Ersser, S. (1991) A search for the therapeutic dimensions of nurse–patient interaction. In: McMahon, R. and Pearson, A. (eds) *Nursing as Therapy* London: Chapman & Hall.

Finch, J. (1986) "It's great to have someone to talk to": the ethics and politics of interviewing women. In Bell, C. and Roberts, H. (eds) *Social Researching: Politics, Problems, Practice*. London: Routledge & Kegan Paul.

Glaser, B. and Strauss, A. (1967) *The Discovery of Grounded Theory: Strategies for Qualitative Research*. Chicago: Aldine.

Gold, R.L. (1958) Roles in sociological fieldwork. *Social Forces*, **36**, 217–223.

Hammersley, M. (1990) *Reading Ethnographic Research: a Critical Guide*. London: Longman.

Hammersley, M. (1992) *What's Wrong With Ethnography? Methodological Explorations*. London: Routledge.

Hammersley, M. and Atkinson, P. (1983) *Ethnography: Principles in Practice* London: Tavistock Publications.

James, N. (1984) A postscript to nursing. In Bell, C. and Roberts, H. (eds) *Social Researching: Politics, Problems, Practice*. London: Routledge & Kegan Paul.

Johnson, J.M. (1975) *Doing Field Research*. New York: Free Press.

Liebow, E. (1967) *Tally's Corner*. London: Routledge & Kegan Paul.

Melia, K. (1987) *Learning and Working: the Occupational Socialisation of Nurses*. London: Tavistock.

Munhall, P. (1988) Ethical considerations in qualitative research. *Western Journal of Nursing Research*, **10**(2), 15–162.

National Institute for Nursing (1993) *Code of Conduct for Researchers*. Oxford: National Institute for Nursing.

Olesen, V.L. and Whittaker, E.W. (1967) Role-making in participant observation: processes in the researcher–actor relationship. *Human Organisation*, **26**, 273–281.

Powdermaker, H. (1966) *Stranger and Friend: the Way of an Anthropologist*. New York: W. Norton & Co.

Punch, M. (1986) *The Politics and Ethics of Fieldwork. Qualitative Research Methods*, 3. Beverly Hills: Sage Publications.

Robinson, C.A. and Thorne, S.E. (1988) Dilemmas of ethics and validity in qualitative nursing research. *The Canadian Journal of Nursing Research*, **20**(1), 65–76.

Rosehan, D.L. (1973) On being sane in insane places. *Science*, **179**, 250–258.

Spradley, J. (1979) *The Ethnographic Interview*. New York: Holt, Rinehart & Winston.

Towell, D. (1975) *Understanding Psychiatric Nursing: a Sociological Study of Modern Psychiatric Nursing Practice*. London: Royal College of Nursing.

Wax, R. (1971) *Doing Fieldwork, Warnings and Advice*. Chicago: University of Chicago Press.

Whyte, W.F. (1981) *Street Corner Society, the Social Culture of an Italian Slum*. Chicago: University of Chicago Press.

Further reading

Hobbs, D. and May, T. (eds) (1993) *Interpreting the Field: Accounts of Ethnography*. Oxford: Oxford University Press.

5

"Watching Me Watching You": Dilemmas in Pain Assessment of Children

Sylvia Buckingham

Introduction

In the autumn of 1990, I undertook a research project as part of the honours component of a degree course. This account is a personal recollection of and reflection on the reality of doing my first research project. In particular I shall try and comment honestly on the ethical dilemmas that I encountered as the project evolved. Most of these situations were uncomfortable for me and I found myself unsure as to how I should handle them. In reality many were over very quickly. None could be said to have been life threatening and had I not been there to observe them, they would most probably have gone unnoticed.

It can be argued that by writing this chapter I am at risk of criticism. Why, some of you may ask did I not take action in certain situations? This, I hope, will become clear as my feelings and the individual circumstances and situations in which the dilemmas arose are explored. I would also argue, perhaps naively, that if we really care about developing nursing, one way of doing so is by being honest with each other. I hope that you will learn something from this that may help, either in your first attempt at research or in the care that you give to your patients. Although this work relates specifically to a project involving children, the dilemmas identified may strike a chord with those of you in other areas of nursing.

Aim of the Project

The aim of the project was to establish what skills and knowledge nurses use when assessing toddlers for pain. The particular group of toddlers I chose were those undergoing day surgery. Given that more children than ever before are receiving treatment on a day case basis and there is limited time to understand individual behaviour, it seemed to me vital to try and identify what elements of nursing skills and knowledge were used when assessing pain. This particular group of children are often deemed to have minimal pain because "they are only day cases".

Pain assessment in children has always been a challenging area for paediatric nurses (McGrath, 1989, 1990; Wallace, 1989, Action for Sick Children, 1993). Numerous factors come into play including developmental differences, previous experience, culture, the effect of anxiety on pain, and even the previous pain experience of the carer. Improved medical and surgical techniques have reduced infant mortality, and there have been huge advances in the treatment of congenital abnormalities and previously fatal illnesses (Brandon, 1986). Curiously, the ability of nurses to assess pain effectively and prescribe the appropriate nursing intervention has remained limited (Wong and Baker, 1988; Wallace, 1989; Carr, 1990; Carpenter, 1990).

I had looked at aspects of pain and its assessment in a previous paper (Buckingham, 1990) and from my clinical experience knew it was an area of care which nurses still found frustrating and where they seemed to possess limited understanding. This is not said as a criticism of nurses but rather as an indication of the complexity of pain and its assessment. It may also be a reflection of how pain is viewed by educationalists. For many years it has been an "add-on" rather than a topic in its own right. I would argue that pain is the common denominator in disease and as such should be considered first in any curriculum. The nurses' response may also be an indictment of the way that pain has been viewed historically by managers. Why is it not at the forefront, when it comes to managing care? Assessment of pain is surely the linchpin upon which the subsequent implementation of nursing care is based. It has major implications for cost-effective care, as all of the activities of daily living must be affected if we are in pain. A client's psychosocial being will not be at peace nor heal as quickly when in pain and yet we remain poor at identifying and actively pursuing pain assessment and its relief.

In 1990, the Royal College of Surgeons issued a report which clearly identified that the management of pain in children was unsatisfactory. Their research revealed that 75% of children were in pain on the day of surgery, 13% in severe pain (RCS, 1990). This document was published at the optimum time for me, as pain assessment was clearly an area in which research was to be of value. I had identified, through a review of the literature, that the toddler age group was lacking in pain assessment research.

Deciding on the Research Methods

I have a passion for my speciality, as many nurses do. Therefore, no amount of work would be too much for me in the attempt to find out more about the way toddlers manifest signs of pain and how this is assessed by nurses. Thus, I chose not to replicate others' work (this was largely because little had been published). Instead, I decided to use three different data collection techniques (triangulation) as I believed that this would yield data that would give me a better understanding of the complexities of the pain assessment process. I believed that by observing the same elements of nursing practice in three different ways, I could truly add to the body of knowledge and make a contribution to nursing. I have since called this the "change the world" syndrome!

Research Design and Data Collection Methods

A review of the literature on research methodology indicated that for the purpose of this study a qualitative, ethnographic approach would be suit-able. Geertz (1973) describes ethnography as a second-order interpretation of actions and people, one with another. I wanted to gain an understanding of how nurses acted with children in specific situations and how nursing knowledge guided their actions with children in pain. In ethnography mul-tiple methods of data collection are used. Thus, I chose to use: participant observation, guided interview and questionnaire. These methods were to yield large quantities of data which, on reflection, were too much for a first-time researcher.

Participant Observation

I purposely chose to observe clinical practice prior to asking respondents to fill out questionnaires and be interviewed. In this way, I thought that I would both minimise bias and enable respondents to reflect on the practice which I had seen as a participant observer. As a paediatric nurse, I felt that I could participate in some clinical work on the ward and be fairly unobtrusive. However, other writers (Nisbet, 1977; Bell, 1987), say that participant observa-tion is not an easy option and that skill is required to identify significant events. As the project unfolded, I wondered whether I was skilled enough.

Leninger (1985) talks about the role of the observer within the social group and the importance of this role in determining what the observer sees. Trust is seen as being vital in order to get "back stage" and learn about the true realities of the group. I had spent 18 months spasmodically visiting the ward to undertake teaching sessions, as part of my degree and also to collect information for course assignments. Data collection for the research took place on two or three days each week over a three-month period. I had worked hard, or so I believed, in gaining trust and acceptance by the staff. How did I know that I was accepted? I took cues from the way I was spoken to and the way that all of the staff included me in discussions. I was also involved with clinical practice and with what was happening to patients in the ward. This involvement and acceptance as one of the team was made very clear to me one day when a child had unexpectedly died. I was asked to sit in with staff and I was the chief tea maker on that day. This I felt clearly identified me as one of them.

This acceptance, however, and becoming "one of the team" may have had a deleterious effect on my ability to observe practice in an unbiased fashion. It also made it much more difficult to intercede in situations where I was unhappy about nursing practice. This friendship led to some agonising ethical dilemmas, which I will consider in more detail later in the chapter.

Critical Incident Technique

As a guide to help me identify specific areas of practice related to pain assessment, I used critical incident technique (Flanagan, 1954) and my own criteria for deciding what constituted a critical incident. This, in turn, I had formulated from previous research on pain assessment in children. Benner (1984, p. 300) is perhaps the most famous nursing exponent of the critical incident technique. She used it to collect direct observations of nursing practice, in such a way as to analyse and more fully understand hitherto unrecognised levels of ability, thereby identifying the transition from novice to expert practitioner.

The Questionnaire

The aim of the questionnaire was to encourage the nurse to reflect on the care given to the toddler and on the particular ways in which pain was considered and assessed. The questionnaire was designed to accommodate Benner's critical incident method and work by Bradshaw and Zeanah (1986) related to pain assessment in children. By using open-ended questions, I knew from the research methods textbooks that I would be giving respondents the opportunity to express situations in their own words. The questionnaire was given to each respondent at the end of the period of observed practice. The respondent was then expected to complete the questionnaire within 24 hours and return it to me.

The Guided Interview

It is said that the guided interview often yields data difficult to collect by any other means. The structure was roughly known, but I had no way of knowing how the respondent would answer. In practice this method worked quite well, but again I was left with a huge amount of data to analyse. I had hoped that all of the methods would combine to reveal new ways of thinking about what nurses do intuitively when assessing pain. I also hoped that the research would elicit the tacit knowledge that is difficult to describe but that drives practice and actions, the "knowing in action" that Schon (1983, p. 25) describes. I wanted to be able to identify and extract this tacit knowledge and ultimately to categorise it. I was aware that all of the respondents in the project were qualified nurses, many with several years of practice behind them. Therefore, I knew that the way in which I pitched and worded the questions was vital, in order not to appear condescending, insulting or irritating to them. I think that this was achieved because of the way we had worked together over the months.

I did not anticipate just how much data this method of interviewing would yield. One 20 minute interview can take three to four hours to transcribe. On reflection, I should have used a structured interview which I could have slotted into easily analysable patterns, which would have yielded quantifiable results. During the data analysis, I realised that I had gathered enough material for numerous projects. This in itself was unsettling and I believe that researchers can go through a period of bereavement whilst discarding data that does not directly relate to the research. No one had told me this and for several days I was confused and unclear as to what to do with such a wealth of information.

Although I had undertaken a small pilot study, the actual project threw up many more queries and situations than I had bargained for. In particular, what to do if the person I had observed was not on duty the next day, having gone off sick or having been put suddenly on to night duty. How could I undertake the interview? Would it mean that they would forget the details of their involvement, if I had to leave it for a few days? This had not been a problem in the pilot study. By leaving a longer period of time between the observation and the interview was I invalidating the project? No matter, the work had to be done. I had a degree to attain and a deadline to meet!

Ethical Considerations Prior to the Project

In the period before I actually undertook the project, I had set out my methods of data collection, reviewed the literature, completed the pilot study and considered the ethics of the work. I was told by the hospital manager that I did not need to take my proposal to the ethics committee, as I was not actually interacting with patients. This was inconsistent with how my seconding health authority would have viewed the proposal. Their policy was to rigorously scrutinise all nursing research proposals for their suitability. This inconsistency left me a little uneasy throughout the data collection period, especially as I discovered that two other research projects (conducted by medical students) were in progress with the same client group. If all research proposals had been through the ethics committee, I suspect that this problem would not have arisen.

My primary concern was for the child and I decided that I must intervene if no other staff recognised that the child was in pain. This honourable decision was to give me numerous calls to question my own and other's practice over the weeks of the observation. To preserve anonymity, the children were assigned a letter of the alphabet, the nurse a number. The staff on the ward were interested in my project and asked me what I was researching. They knew that I would be observing their clinical practice and had given their consent but they were not aware of my specific focus. I felt guilty and almost deceitful that, prior to the observation period, I did not explain exactly what I would be looking for. My feelings of guilt were heightened during the data collection when I observed poor practice. Should I have been more explicit about my work and if I had, would they have been so eager to participate?

Ethical Dilemmas

Example one

- The child was crying and the nurse spoke generally with an: "Oh, she's off!" but did not move from the nursing station to investigate why the child was crying. The parents were present and they were left to manage. It was clear to me that they were unsure what the problem was. Soon after this the child wet the bed and I surmised that the child may have been either in pain or discomfort from her operation or because she wanted to go to the toilet. If the child had wanted to go to the toilet why had the parents not realised this?

Some people may think it reasonable to leave parents to manage; however, the child had recently returned from theatre following surgery. I had the knowledge from my literature review, that parents often cannot manage the care required by their children in hospital for a variety of reasons (Copp, 1985). From my point of view, I felt that the parents may not have felt able to say: "Nurse, come and take over. I do not know why my child is crying." This is the feeling I had while watching the non-verbal cues of the mother and father, as they sat by the girl's bedside. I felt angry that the nurse did not intercede and help the child. I wanted to say something but what would happen if I did? Would the nurse take offence and consider that I was interfering in her care? How could I explain my concerns, how long would it take? The nurse was very busy writing the discharge papers. This was probably her main reason for not attending to the child. Would an interchange between us change her practice, or would I simply be viewed with suspicion? Would she withdraw from the research project and leave me with fewer subjects? Would she tell her colleagues and undermine their confidence in me? Would this lead to them all withdrawing from the project? But did I not have more knowledge because I had reviewed the literature concerning the role of parents of children in hospital? What rights did I really have as a visitor on her ward?

The role of the parent

When a child is admitted to hospital, I believe that the role of the parents is much more complex than originally thought. It may be that the parents have never seen their child suffering in this way and find it difficult to cope themselves, let alone be able to help their child. It may remind the parents of their own experiences in hospital. A relative may have recently been hospitalised or even died in hospital. It may be that the parents have an expectation that the nurses will "do the nursing" when the child is sick. The concept of partnership in care is one that nurses have but one wonders how often this is shared with the family, in a way that they can understand.

It has been fashionable for paediatric nurses to believe that the concept of partnership in care is fundamental for the good of the patient: that family participation will ensure that the amount of anxiety suffered by the child will be minimised because the family are involved. In general and at a superficial level, this may well be true but if we look closely at individual needs, fears and beliefs it may be that every child and family unit has to be individually assessed for their ability to cope with hospitalisation and the role that they wish to play in this. I believe that ground rules should be set by the nurse caring for each child. The family members must be clear that they play the role that they choose to, rather than the role nurses think is appropriate.

The care of children admitted for day surgery is particularly complex as relationships and understandings have to be formed in a very short space of time. Nursing expertise is essential to give the level of care required to achieve a positive experience for each child admitted. In the case of the child described, no relationship had developed between the parents, child and nurse assigned to them, no ground rules had been set and no common understandings about roles had been agreed. This was a frequent conclusion I came to while witnessing the interactions of many nurses, parents and children during the participant observation period.

Where did I fit in to all this? I felt unhappy and uncomfortable in my own role as participant observer. Did I get on with the menial tasks I had allocated myself to do or did I discuss the thoughts and feelings that I had? In the event I did nothing. I wonder now if this is the reason that these few minutes of observed nursing practice are still so fresh in my mind. I also wonder whether the uncomfortable feelings I had originally, feel as strong now because I never resolved them at the time. Did I let the child and family down by not interceding? I felt that I had not lived up to my own personal ethics, or had I?

Example two

In this example, one particular child demonstrated various behaviours which I, as the observer, noted and translated into different meanings. The first incident took place as follows.

- The child was unhappy and irritable, his mother had lifted him out of the bed on to the floor. The nurse asked the mother specifically if she thought that the child was in pain. The mother replied that she thought that he was irritable but not in pain.

My concern over this specific incident was that the child had had an epidural anaesthetic during the operation procedure. Was the child fully aware of the sensations in his legs? Could his legs function normally? Was he afraid? How much could he comprehend about the situation? How much had the mother been told and what had she told the child? I was frustrated because I could not answer any of these questions.

The second and third incidents were as follows.

- The child was becoming restless and irritable. The nurse took and recorded his vital signs and then told the mother that he could have a drink. No notice was taken of the child's behaviour.
- The child appeared pale and was shuddering. The mother requested that the child be given toast (if toast and drink were tolerated, they could go home). The nurse asked the child if he would like something to eat but he did not reply. Shortly after this the child vomited.

According to the Bradshaw and Zeanah's (1986) categories, which I was using as an objective analysis of pain, this child was clearly demonstrating pain behaviours. The mother was extremely anxious and when I looked at the child's notes I discovered that this child had been born prematurely and had spent several weeks in the neonatal unit. He had been very sick. I wondered whether this was the reason for the mother bringing with her, her own mother and a sibling to the ward for the day. In many ways, it surely would have been easier for her to have asked her mother to care for the other child away from the stresses of a hospital environment. Was it necessary then, for her to bring them for her own support? As I observed this family, it struck me that the mother was extremely anxious and that much of her anxiety was possibly being transferred to the child. As it was not within my remit nor my research proposal to pursue this area any further, I could only make assumptions about the mother's reasons for her behaviour and the way her concerns were transferred to the child.

However, it is interesting to note that the nurse asked specifically if the child was in pain and the mother denied that he was. Although the nurse said afterwards that she was aware of the child's behaviour, she allowed the mother to decide. This observation brings in to question the parents' ability to assess their own child for pain. The influences of the child's previous medical history can only be surmised. It raises the question, at what point do nurses take over and act for the child, rather than rely on parents? Parental anxiety and the expectations nurses have of parents' ability when a child is hospitalised have been mentioned previously, but this extract again high-lights the complexity of the topic and the need for nurses to consider all aspects of the child's current and previous medical history, prior to making any assessments. It also identifies the importance of establishing an open relationship with the family as early as possible. Perhaps the most important aspect is the influence that previous hospital admissions have on future behaviours. The responsibility for ensuring that each hospital admission is as positive as possible, lies partly with nurses. If this process is relegated to ancillary staff or seen as a non-nursing duty and is viewed as a negative experience by the child and family, it may have possible consequences for the rest of the child's life.

In this example I had a greater knowledge of the child and his previous medical history than the nurse caring for him. I wanted to challenge her on the way that she had allowed the mother to make the decisions regarding the child's pain. However, in her view, which is reinforced by the general concept of family centred care, the nurse had taken the appropriate action by asking the mother if she thought the child was in pain. It was my greater knowledge gained from the literature review and the child's notes that made me question her practice. It was not fair to the nurse if I intervened, but was it fair to the child? I could have shared my knowledge with the nurse but there was no time for this, given the reality of the ward environment and the nurse's workload.

Example three

The interactions observed with this third child and the nurse were very brief.

- The nurse commented to the mother on bringing the child back from theatre that he was very cute and lovely and settled. From my viewpoint the child was settled but very pale. This child was much more difficult to observe because he was in a cubicle. I could only observe interactions by contriving to be near to the door or window of the cubicle, which was not easy. Again, this problem had not been experienced during the pilot study. The parents commented later in the morning to me that they thought that he had had painful "twinges". However, the nurse thought that the child was settled every time she saw him. In this observation there was no interaction with the family at all. At no time were their opinions or comments sought. As the morning went on the child was seen to be holding himself more stiffly but mum said that she thought that he was not too bad, considering what he had gone through.

In this example there was a complete contradiction between what I observed and what the nurse saw. She was extremely busy with the theatre list and looked in to see this child on an *ad hoc* basis. Other nurses undertook some of the observations and documented his vital signs. The mother thought that the child had some small degree of pain but this, she felt, was expected, given that he had had surgery. This left me feeling very unsure of what my action should be. I reminded myself why I was doing the study: to identify what skills and knowledge nurses use to assess toddlers for pain. The nurse was using visual observation skills based on her knowledge of children. In her opinion the child did not appear to be in pain. The mother was unsure about the degree of pain which was acceptable. The cues were very difficult to decipher at times and many were extremely brief and subtle. Again, I felt that my greater "insider" knowledge was working against me. Should I intervene or should I allow the nurse to decide? In the event I let the nurse continue. Something that the child said later in the day made me question this decision. He said that he did not want "to go on holiday again". I suspect that he had been told that he was coming into hospital with his suitcase and this was "like going on holiday". He was being given the idea that this was to be a good experience. Again, I can only suspect that the child had a very unhappy experience. His pain was not identified by the nurse. His mother commented to the effect that he should expect some degree of pain. This highlights for me the belief held by some people that pain is to be expected and has to be tolerated. That was perhaps, a reason why no comments were made to the nurse regarding the child's pain nor any pain relief sought. Reflecting on the role of the parent, this situation again underlines the complexity of this role and the different health beliefs held by individual families.

On a busy surgical ward, nurses are always pushed for time and staff rarely use pain assessment tools. This was the reason I was undertaking the research project, to try and gain a clearer picture of what was considered helpful when assessing toddlers for pain. I was also learning about factors which affected the pain assessment process. However, the dilemmas I felt were something I had not been prepared for and I had very few people I could turn to for advice. This in itself was revealing, as part of me was afraid to discuss my worries in case I was subsequently told that I should have acted, instead of leaving the judgements to the nurses I was observing. I tried to comfort myself by thinking of other researchers who had had dilemmas. In particular, I remembered the Robertsons who undertook some very harrowing research in the 1950s (Robertson, 1958). Part of the Robertsons' research involved making films of children being admitted to hospital and left without parents. This husband and wife research team had many heart rending moments during the months of observation, but the research changed practice and ultimately was worth the trauma. I too wanted my project to actually make a difference to clinical practice.

This last statement may seem either very grand or particularly naive when we consider that the topic area being studied was pain and as I have discussed earlier, it is a very complex and difficult area. However, what I thought I would be observing would be clinical practice which would reveal how nurses use a variety of skills and knowledge to undertake pain assessment in toddlers. I did not realise, and neither did my small pilot study show, that in reality what I would be observing would be something less than this. On reflection perhaps, what I wanted to observe was practice as I wanted it to be, rather than how it was. This I had not thought about and I wonder whether this was a further reason for my feeling uncomfortable in my role.

However, a further observation clearly showed what I judged to be good nursing practice. It also manifested the use of skills and knowledge to their full effect.

Example four

- The nurse gave the mother a detailed account of the process of recovery the child would undergo during the day. Post-operative needs were discussed, as was the analgesia that the child had received in theatre. The side-effects of medications were also identified and discussed. The nurse then clarified with the child and mother that should they feel he was in pain, then more analgesia could and would be given. The nurse then explained that she too would be observing him.
- The nurse kept a close eye on this child despite other children to care for. On one occasion the mother had left the ward and the child woke up. The nurse watched him and he settled with no obvious sign of pain. When the mother returned to the ward the nurse immediately informed the mother of what had happened. Later in the morning the nurse went to the child and asked the mother if she felt that the child was "OK". During this conversation the nurse was watching the child and she lifted the bedclothes

in order to observe the child's wound. Throughout this, the child remained asleep on his stomach.

In the questionnaire the nurse identified that she has used visual observation and vital signs as a means of assessing the child for pain. The child did not demonstrate any signs of pain during his recovery period; however, this had not prevented the nurse from undertaking regular and detailed observations of his behaviour. The nurse had filled out a detailed care plan for this child, in which there was more detail than I had seen previously for the day case children. She was working with a student nurse on this shift. I wondered if this had had any influence on the amount of detail documented and the time spent with the mother. If this was the case then she was providing a very good role model for the student.

This nurse was very aware of the behaviours of the children in her care and went to them on a regular basis. Her workload was no less than on previous occasions when other nurses had been observed. This nurse was clearly working from a good knowledge base and it was this that I had hoped to capture in the research.

During the remainder of the participant observation period, I continued to observe differences in the way nurses assessed for pain behaviours. What began to emerge was the most difficult dilemma of all for me personally and one that I was not sure how to resolve or indeed discuss. What emerged was that there was clearly a difference between the way that paediatric-and non-paediatric-trained nurses used their skills and knowledge to assess for pain.

I had identified children who appeared to me to be manifesting pain behaviours, yet several incidents were observed where no action was taken by the nurse. It became increasingly apparent that the amount of positive nursing action undertaken with the toddler and parent was greater if the nurse was paediatric-trained. The other (non-paediatric-trained) nursing group consisted of enrolled nurses. The guided interviews revealed an equal knowledge by both groups of a broad range of pain behaviours appropriate to toddlers. An underlying theme which therefore emerged was one of a theory–practice gap, which I believe to have been related to a deficit in the ability to apply theory to practice and reflect on practice. Was it the case that enrolled nurses were unable to synthesise the knowledge they had acquired into clinical practice? This emerging pattern was extremely difficult for me to divulge. I wanted to feed back the results of the project to the staff. The reason for doing it had been to help develop a pain assessment tool for toddlers. How then, could I reveal that there was this clear difference in the groups of nurses observed?

The enrolled nurses in the project had been much more concerned with filling out the documentation and getting the job done compared to the paediatric nurses who had been more concerned with giving detailed care.

The different groups used the time they had available to different ends. This could be said to reflect directly the way that the two different groups had been educated and trained. By identifying this difference, I was possibly creating a problem for the ward and the hospital as a whole. I was also betraying the trust and friendship given to me by the nurses in this ward area.

My decision was to reduce the amount of discussion related to the differences in the groups to a minimum and to concentrate on the information I had gained on pain assessment. The underlying theme of differences within the groups of nurses was not what I had set out to establish. What I had to concentrate on was the skills and knowledge that were used by this group of nurses when assessing toddlers for pain.

It has been argued earlier in this chapter that children being admitted for day care require a greater understanding (Taylor, 1983). This need for understanding applies also to the child's relatives. Throughout the data collection period of my research project, I came across the dilemmas that I have tried to share with you. There is no criticism intended of the group of enrolled nurses with whom I worked, rather I am concerned that we expect too much of staff who are provided with little or no continuing development, to enable them to meet changing needs.

The assessment of pain in toddlers is a complex issue. The research clearly identified this. I gained some insight into the skills and knowledge that were used in the pain assessment process and I came to reconsider the role of the family and the manner in which nurses undertake pain assessment. I have tried to put this information to good use during my teaching of pain and pain assessment, to staff and students. As I stated at the beginning of this chapter, I was extremely naive when I began the project. I wanted to change the world. I did not, but what I did find were numerous dilemmas that I had not anticipated. I have written about a very personal part of my professional life, and I hope that by sharing this account with you it has in some way given you a greater understanding of the reality of ethical dilemmas in research.

References

Action for Sick Children (1993) Managing pain in children. *Nursing Standard Special Supplement*, **7**(25), 10 March.

Bell, J. (1987) *Doing Your Research Project*. Oxford University Press.

Benner, P. (1984) *From Novice To Expert. Excellence and Power in Clinical Nursing*. Addison Wesley.

Bradshaw, C. and Zeanah, P. (1986) Paediatric nurse's assessment of pain in children. *Journal of Paediatric Nursing*, **1**, 314–322.

Brandon, S. (1986) *Children in Hospital*. London: National Association of Children in Hospital.

Buckingham, S. (1990) Situational analysis; the assessment of paediatric pain in a surgical ward. How do qualified nurses assess . . . how do students learn? Unpublished Paper.

Carpenter, P. (1990) New methods for assessing young children's self-report of fear of pain. *Journal of Pain and Symptom Management*, **5**(4), 233–240.

Carr, E. (1990) Post-operative pain; patient's expectations and experiences. *Journal of Advanced Nursing*, **15**, 89–100.

Copp, L. (1985) *Perspectives on Pain; Recent Advances in Nursing*. London: Churchill Livingstone.

Flanagan, J. (1954) The critical incident technique, *Psychological Bulletin*, **51**, 327–358.

Geertz, C. (1973) *The Interpretation of Cultures*. New York: Basic Books.

Leninger, M. (1985) *Qualitative Research Methods in Nursing*. New York: Saunders Co.

McGrath, D.P. (1989) Evaluating a child's pain. *Journal of Pain and Symptom Management*, **4**(4), 198–214.

McGrath, D.P. (1990) *Pain in Children*. London: Guildford Press.

McGrath, D.P. and Craig, K. (1989) Developmental and psychological factors in children's pain. *Acute Pain in Children, Pediatric Clinical of North America*, **36**(4), 823–835.

Nisbet, J.D. (1977) Small scale research; guidelines and suggestions for development. *Scottish Educational Studies*, **9** (May), 13–17.

RCS (1990) *Report of The Working Party; Pain After Surgery*. London: Royal College of Surgeons and Anaesthetists.

Robertson, J. (1958) *Young Children in Hospital*. London: Tavistock.

Schon, D.A. (1983) *The Reflective Practitioner, How Professionals Think in Action*. New York: Basic Books.

Taylor, P. (1983) Post operative pain in toddler and preschoolage children. *Maternal Child Nursing Journal*, **12**(1), 35–50.

Wallace, M. (1989) Temperament, a variable in children's pain management. *Pediatric Nursing*, **15**(2), 118–121.

Wong, D. and Baker, C. (1988) Pain in children: comparison of assessment scales. *Pediatric Nursing*, Jan./Feb., Vol. 14, No. 1, pp. 8–17.

6

Research in Psychiatric Settings: Some Ethical Issues

Kim Lützén

Introduction

The aim of this chapter is to illuminate some ethical issues encountered during six weeks of field research on a psychiatric ward in Sweden using the grounded theory method.

At the planning stage of the study, my own practical experience as a psychiatric nurse was chiefly history. Nevertheless, I had always felt a nagging ambition to explore, in a more objective way, the everyday reality of nurses in psychiatric settings. Underlying this goal were the many myths and misconceptions held by lay people *and* other professionals outside the field of psychiatry concerning mental illness and the institutional setting. For instance, a common remark is that persons who work in psychiatry must be a little mad themselves!

The practice of psychiatric nursing has undergone many changes through the years, accommodating various conceptions of mental illness and treatment modes. Alongside having to adjust to the different definitions of mental illness, the psychiatric nurse is not always clear about her role because nurses are often faced with situations where they are expected to control or modify patients' behaviour. This can result in feelings of conflict between the "caring" role and the "custodial" role. Moreover, taking care of persons who refuse treatment often results in an emotional upheaval and feelings of defeat among the staff. My own experience left me with many unanswered questions, and one in particular was: why do nurses choose to work in psychiatry? This background was the catalyst for research that gave me new and unanticipated insights into the moral nature of the nurse–patient interaction (Lützén, 1993).

As I will hope to convey by this chapter, the choice of a qualitative research approach in itself raises ethical issues which need to be dealt with in a candid way. These questions concern not only the emerging *ethical* perspective of the nurse–patient relationship but also the ethical *issues* concerning the formulation of the research problem, design, data-collection and publication of results.

I will first give a brief description of the context in which the research took place. This will involve addressing those attributes of psychiatry and psychiatric nursing which can be viewed as "moral". These attributes can be defined as moral because they relate to a practice of medicine that often has to do with restricting individual freedom according to best interest standards. On a conceptual level, ethics in psychiatry often concerns the relationship between paternalism and freedom of choice. On a practical level, ethics in psychiatry concerns the justification of different means of limiting freedom of choice, for example, keeping some people behind locked doors.

I will continue by identifying some of the problems that arose during the major phases of the research and discuss why I view these to be ethical issues. In conclusion, after reflecting on this experience, I shall summarise some points as recommendations for similar fieldwork in the future.

Moral Attributes of Psychiatry

Since the establishment of psychiatry as a branch of medicine in the western world, the incarceration of the mentally ill has been the subject of much ideological controversy. No other area of medicine is divided to the same extent by different ideologies and theoretical perspectives. A recent example taken from forensic psychiatry illustrates this point. Six experts were called upon to determine whether a particularly violent murder was an act of insanity or not. Three of these psychiatric experts firmly claimed that the accused person was not mentally ill at the time. The other experts, equally convinced by their examination of the person, believed that he was mentally ill. In the latter case it would then follow that he would not be held "legally" responsible in the same way as a person who is not mentally ill would be. Similar disputes, although not quite so dramatic, demonstrate that the concept of normality cannot be scientifically defined and agreed upon within the discipline of psychiatry in the same way as, for example, hepatitis can be.

Social ideals and values determine, as well as limit, the distribution of psychiatric care and treatment. As such, a person's need for psychiatric care is to a large extent dependent on attitudes towards and evaluations of the vital goals of man. Moreover, these goals are culturally determined and vary from one society to another (Nordenfelt, 1987). With regard to ideas and perceptions concerning mental illness, each society has its own way of appraising human behaviour and deciding where the boundaries go for what is normal and abnormal (Sachs and Krantz, 1991).

Peter Miller (Rose and Miller, 1986) points out that critiques of psychiatry date almost from its inception and have had an important function in the development and modernisation of psychiatry. Most important is the critique of the asylum, for example, Erving Goffman's (1959, 1961), field research and essays on the social situation of mental patients.

Alongside the juridical critique of psychiatry that concerns the rights of patients, there was also critique directed towards the theoretical explanations of mental illness. The anti-psychiatry movement in the 1960s was characterised by the epistemological assertion that mental illness did not exist, either as an objective phenomenon or as an illness that could be medically treated (Rose and Miller, 1986). Thus, not only has critique focused on psychiatric institutions but also on the concept of madness itself. Definitions of madness are linked to the treatment.

The whole range of psychiatric treatments, for example, electroconvulsive shock therapy and psychotropic medication, was considered repressive. But compared to locked doors and physical restraints, these were more sophisticated means of limiting a person's freedom.

It is well documented that the predominant treatment ideology today varies from one psychiatric institution or community mental health service to another. However, there is one axiom that can be named universal: ideological convictions (ideas underpinning theoretical frameworks for aetiology and treatment of mental illness) in psychiatry generate (moral) rules for practice (Strauss et al., 1981). These moral rules are revealed in paternalistic responses aimed at normalising the behaviour of others.

Perhaps the de-institutionalisation movement is in part a consequence of sociological research of psychiatric practice from an "insider's" perspective. Erving Goffman's (1961) fieldwork, for example, provided empirical evidence and arguments concerning the negative effects of institutional life, especially the loss of personal autonomy. Although Goffman did not apply a standard research design or theory that could be tested, his ideas on institutional life and the social organisation of the mental hospital have become well known.

It may be that the trend of "western liberal philosophy", with its emphasis on freedom of choice, paved the way for a whole range of therapies, such as sensitivity training, gestalt therapy, primal therapy and reality therapy, as alternatives o traditional treatment, for example drugs. What these so-called dynamic therapies have in common is that the "client" is urged to be an active rather than a passive participant in his or her own treatment. Thus, the principle of autonomy, meaning self-choice and self-determination, becomes important in a therapeutic sense.

Psychiatry deals with the organic, the functional, i.e. individual psychological awareness, and the social. All of these levels involve their own conceptions of normality and abnormality. The move from asylums and custodial care to community psychiatry and rehabilitation can be interpreted as embracing a more humanitarian and holistic view of the person. Given current realities, this may be an idealistic view not seen in practice.

However, even if there has been a shift from institutional care to rehabilitation and integration in the community, the organisational changes which have taken place do not mean that mental illness has been redefined. Psychiatry continues to exert behavioural control even outside institutional walls (a good example is the dispensing of lithium). Moreover, the availability of minor tranquillisers means that not only are severe psychotic disorders treated but also a variety of psychosocial problems can be dealt with on a community basis.

Psychiatric Nursing

Social change and advances made in psychiatry created a need for establishing disciplinary specialities outside medicine itself, for example nursing. This meant that the type of nursing required changed from custodial to therapeutic. As a substantial amount of literature shows, the nurse gained significance not only as a therapeutic agent, but also as someone who was, and still is, in the position to know the patient best. This is mainly because it is the nurse who spends consistently the most amount of time with the patient.

Currently, the existence of distinctly different theoretical perspectives and levels of knowledge means also that the type of professional commitment to the patient varies among nurses. Many nurse theorists emphasise the importance of the therapeutic relationship in the process of the patient's recovery. However, acting as a therapeutic agent also means that dealing with problems such as aggression, violence and refusing medication and treatment always includes a moral component.

The moral nature of psychiatric practice cannot be supplanted by any organisational or structural changes. Nurses, because of their closeness to the patient on an everyday basis, often claim to *know* the patient's needs best, even if these are not expressed by the patient himself or herself. When the patient lacks motivation, insight or cognitive ability to make their own decisions concerning daily care, the nurse is morally committed to intervene.

Moreover, defining the role of the psychiatric nurse as a *therapist*, may imply that nursing *care* is not therapeutic or that care and therapy may be perceived as mutually exclusive. Thus, it may be that nurses who have acquired competency in psychotherapeutic skills are uncertain whether their allegiance is to medicine, psychology or nursing.

The core of the above overview is that while psychiatric nursing can theoretically be defined in many ways, how nurses in specific historical, moral and cultural contexts perceive their work must be explored empirically. The conceptual understanding of mental illness and corresponding treatments remains an ethical as well as a scientific question. The role of research in psychiatry is not only aimed at developing medical knowledge, but also at identifying interpersonal aspects that influence patients' well-being.

The institutional setting has primarily been an object of research for social scientists who focus their attention on groups and especially deviant behaviour (Lee, 1993). The systematic enquiry of social research using the grounded theory method introduced by Glaser and Strauss (1967), has been adopted by nurse-researchers to study communication and interactions between staff and patients, particularly in the psychiatric setting (Bunch, 1983).

Formulating the Research Question

Two questions were posed at the outset of the study: can this study be justified in terms of knowledge gained and is all knowledge useful knowledge? Neither of these questions could clearly be answered since the research method chosen meant that not all knowledge gained could be anticipated in the same way as in hypothesis testing.

Lee (1993) points out that it is typical for field research that the focus for research emerges only after data collection has begun. Moreover, qualitative research is still unfamiliar to ethical review committees who evaluate research proposals according to traditional research methods in which all steps, including the anticipated outcome, are known. This meant that my research proposal needed to be carefully written to encompass eventual modifications. For example, in a traditional research proposal, the sample size is known or estimated and is greater than in qualitative research. Therefore an explanation needed to be written into the proposal: firstly, that the strategy of participant observation would generate a substantial amount of data and, secondly, that the focus was on situations and not persons, thus an exact "number" could not be given.

Having the *nurse–patient relationship* as a frame of reference meant that the aim of the research was to develop knowledge about this relationship. As pointed out, the formulation of the research problem had a given ethical dimension. The interpersonal orientation of the research had to be defined as a sensitive topic because it was to do with the exploration of values, feelings, experiential meanings and opinions. Publishing these subjective aspects could have had direct implications for the participants of the study (i.e. nurses) and indirect ones for the patients.

As mentioned above, the aim was to conceptualise essential aspects of psychiatric nursing within the framework of the nurse–patient relationship, from the perspective of nurses. Since psychiatric nursing has few middle-range or substantive theories that can be used to examine or explain the everyday realities of nurse–patient interactions, a qualitative research method for theory-generating aimed at identifying core concepts and their relationship to each other was chosen. Another aim was to generate future research questions from the concepts identified.

A field approach made it possible to observe as well as to interview nurses in the natural setting. As the study progressed, questions concerning the moral dimension of psychiatric nursing evolved:

- What is the moral meaning of the nurse–patient relationship from the perspective of the nurse?
- How can the subjective experience of *moral decision making* in psychiatric nursing be conceptualised?
- How does the individual nurse know what action to take in concrete moral conflicts and how does the nurse justify these actions?

Gaining Entrance

The first phase of fieldwork involves careful preparation in order to gain entrance, i.e. negotiating access to the field where participant observation will be conducted. Since fieldwork implies intrusion, establishing initial contacts and obtaining participant consent to do the research will help to minimise the effects of invasion (Evaneshko, 1985).

There are no specific rules but some general guidelines used by anthropologists can be of help. These include informing the participants of confidentiality and their rights to refuse to participate in the study. Compared to other research strategies, the participants are not anonymous and thus the research may have undesirable effects on the people being studied. As Becker *et al.* (1968) explained:

> . . . participant observation is a process in which the observer's presence in a social situation is maintained for the purpose of scientific investigation. The observer is in a *face-to-face* relationship with the observed and, by participating with them, gathers data.

Since the goal of fieldwork is to "get to know" people in their social (or work life) the researcher embarking upon participant observation must be prepared for voiced objections. If anyone had refused to participate in my study, I was prepared to reconsider other options than observation since it would be impossible to include some and not others in my field of vision.

The main purpose of using the participant observation strategy is to study interactions in the natural setting and to gain an understanding of a phenom-enon from an "insider's" perspective (Schatzman and Strauss, 1973). For this reason, field research can create problems not anticipated in the proposal. Obtaining consent is not always a guarantee that "good" research will be conducted. This is especially so if consent is given by a research ethics committee who is unfamiliar with qualitative research and the impact it has on the people involved in the study.

One of my first tasks was to select a setting that would be suitable for the research, and where I would find nurses from whom I could learn. The ward I selected was located in a mental institution that now does not exist (as a result of the process of de-institutionalisation). In order to minimise any preconceptions and biases, it was important to select a ward where I did not previously know any of the staff or patients. The only person I was acquainted with was one of my thesis advisers who was also chief physician. The staff worked in teams consisting of psychiatrists, social worker, psychologist, registered nurses and mental health care workers (enrolled nurses specialised in psychiatric care). Only the nursing staff wore white uniforms. The ward was categorised as an "open ward" which in theory meant that the door should not be locked.

Although I was a novice researcher, I was aware of the ethical implications of other issues not included in the research proposal and I realised the power of the position I would be in. There was a potential risk that I would be observing activities and practices that could be interpreted as morally unac-ceptable, such as abusive behaviour. Following the advice of more experi-enced field researchers, I met with the staff several times in order to be trusted as a researcher and to negotiate the terms of my presence on the ward. Although the invitation had gone out to all team members, there were a number of people who did not come, or people whose significance I had overlooked (e.g. psychologists and other paramedical staff) and thus not invited. In my eagerness to inform the nursing staff, I had made my first mistake.

Since I was a doctoral student at the time and doing research that was still unconventional for a nurse, gaining entrance to the ward was very much in the hands of the staff. In meeting with the staff, it was important for me to give as much information as possible about the purpose of the study, about how I was going to collect data and about what I would do with my findings. It was mutually decided that I would avoid any interac-tion with the patients in the ward, in order to minimise the potential problem of "role conflict". Although no questions were spontaneously raised about publication, I believed it necessary to anticipate the participants' worry about how the research results would be used. I assured them that the data collected were not going to be used by the administration for the evaluation of staff performance.

Collection of Data and the Emergence of the Moral Dimension of Psychiatric Nursing

The method of grounded theory provided a structure for the simultaneous collection and analysis of data. In brief, theory describing a process or interaction is generated from constant comparative analysis of data obtained by observing and listening. This involves comparing each event with other events and coding these events. Then codes are subsumed into concepts or categories and compared with other categories. The emerging categories give direction to further sampling of events until the point of saturation, i.e. no new observations are made. By using this strategy the generated theory is validated by its close linkage to concrete observations. If the theory is closely linked to data, the researcher will recognise and understand the connection between theory and practice. Although some identical and some different events would become data for other field observers, a generated theory should help to explain common experiences (Schatzman and Strauss, 1973). Other research methods would have to be used to test the theory.

In the attempt to establish and maintain methodological rigour and ana-lytic precision, all my observations, interviews and conversations were documented in field notes or audiotaped (Schatzman and Strauss, 1973). The staff were told that they could read my observational notes at any time. Since the interviews were more personal, the transcriptions were kept con-fidential. (Only once did a nurse ask if she could read my observational notes, and after reading these made no comments.)

While collecting data it was necessary to apply the phenomenological method of "bracketing" or holding in abeyance previous knowledge and reactions (Giorgi, 1985). Two situations can be used to exemplify the need for bracketing.

The first incident occurred during a team conference during which I silently observed and listened to the plans made for patients. When the team's discussion centred around a particular patient, who was well known by all staff because of repeated admissions and for not being "motivated", a nurse said something demeaning about this patient and everyone laughed. I reacted by passing judgement (not voiced) on the staff and in doing so made another mistake – not maintaining my research role and "going native" (i.e. integrating the group's values and norms within my own value system). When I later read my notes I realised how easily a bias can be incorporated into the analysis of data. Value judgements cannot be avoided, but bracketing gave me insight into this during the analysis of data.

The second incident, observed several times during the whole period of fieldwork, was the periodic locking of the door to the ward. The nursing staff justified this action by explaining it was in the best interests of *some* of the patients or as being necessary to prevent a particular patient from leaving. It was not difficult to see the moral implication of this action. Although the purpose was to protect one particular patient from harm (which could be legally justified according to the Mental Health Act), the action also had the effect that it restricted the freedom of other patients who were admitted to the ward on a "voluntary" basis. The question was, did I have a moral responsibility to point out this discrepancy or could I justify being silent?

The above situations are examples of how bracketing has an ethical dimension. Holding values in suspension can also result in non-action in situations where one should ethically intervene. In the first situation my reaction can be seen as moralising, and as not particularly successful bracketing. In the second situation, I faced a choice either to bring to attention and discussion the contradiction implied by the practice of locking doors or to let it go. Both situations can be viewed as methodological problems but they are also ethical problems because only I could decide what to do with my observations. Lincoln and Guba (1985) point out that the very openness of fieldwork and the emergent nature of its design may give rise to the charge that what is included or excluded is entirely a matter of the researcher's own choices. Compared to scientific control, where one manipulates or holds specific variables constant under experimental conditions, qualitative research relies on personal restraint and integrity which means that the field researcher can omit information, leading to inaccurate data.

The above situation, if taken out of context, could be misinterpreted because certain information would be lacking. However, as a field researcher (and as a psychiatric nurse) I had a contextual understanding of the action, mainly because I followed (i.e. listened to and observed) the staff's process of reasoning and concluded that locking the doors was the best alternative and not the result of any arbitrary decision.

The moral dimension of psychiatric nursing was substantiated by actions taken that limited the patients' autonomy. Limiting autonomy was explicitly expressed, for example, locking the door to the ward. Other actions were more subtle, for example, establishing rules that made the patients dependent on the nursing staff. An illustration of this was keeping the patients' cigarettes locked up in the nursing office.

During my fieldwork I also witnessed the dramatic situation of a patient being given an injection by force. This observation was followed up in individual face-to-face interviews. The nurse expressed negative feelings towards coercion and threat of coercion but said that at times these methods were necessary as "a last resort".

The moral aspect of nursing presented itself mainly in the contradictions between what nurses thought *should* be done (ideals) and what *was* actually done in practice. "It is important that the patients participate in their care" is often cited as a nursing ideal, one that I heard repeatedly during my fieldwork. But it was not always easy to maintain this ideal, as in the following example: I observed that patients hung up towels or garments to cover the windows in the doors to their rooms. The nursing staff would come along and consistently remove them. When asked about this, one of the nurses explained: "We need to have a clear view to see that the patient is still breathing".

Other observations led to the conceptualisation "following the unwritten rules". This meant that there was a tacit understanding among the staff that some written rules could be broken in special circumstances, for example, physically restraining a patient until the doctor comes. Other types of unwritten rules have to do with patient approach. One example is taken from a team meeting and, as is the practice, patients were not included. There was a knock on the door but it was ignored. The staff exchanged glances with one another and one nurse said: "It is a patient" – but did not get up to find out what this patient wanted. The meeting continued as if nothing had happened. It is an unwritten rule that patients are not allowed to interrupt staff meetings.

All instances of "following the unwritten rules" were justified in the name of "good" actions in the best interests or safety of the patient. However, some of the nurses believed that restricting patients' autonomy was an outcome of the organisation of the hospital, for example, lack of staff created an unsafe climate for the patients and the nursing staff felt compelled to lock the door. The nurses believed that organisational shortcomings reflected an ideology that was different from their own, leaving few behavioural options.

However, enhancing or limiting the patient's autonomy often depended on the individual nurse's interpretation of the patient's immediate needs. Following the unwritten rules created a group alliance among the nursing staff which was essential to deal with the tensions that resulted from the experienced *ideological conflicts*.

The concept "ideology", as it emerged in this study, was defined as opinions and norms related to the aims and functions of the nursing staff, medical staff and hospital organisation. Although the institutional ideology may promote ideas and purposes for care, it was not the aim of this study to compare ideologies. In this study, the use of the term "ideology" was defined as the ideals about psychiatric nursing, its aims and methods, as perceived by the nurses. These ideals determined the written and unwritten rules of practice. In consequence, the ideological *conflict* was believed to originate in the different moral imperatives imposed by structural requirements on the one hand and personal and professional ideals of nursing care on the other. Disparate "oughts" were difficult to put into practice because of (perceived) ideological differences.

Implications for the Psychiatric Patient

The patient is in a vulnerable position, dependent on others for his or her daily needs. In cases where paternalism can be justified, it is important that decisions are not made in the interests of private intentions. In reference to this research, permission to conduct the study was not obtained from the patients. However, information *about* the patients and all forms of interaction with the patients could not be avoided. For example, when I sat and wrote my field notes in the nursing office, patients would come and ask me certain questions. I could not pretend I did not see them, nor could I ignore the more simple questions, such as asking the time or what my name was. The agreement with the staff was that I would not use any patient information in my written report.

This study, identifying the moral aspect of nursing, provided a framework for continued research focusing on moral decision-making in psychiatric nursing practice. However, one could ask, what use is this knowledge if psychiatric patients and their experiences are not included? If we can accept the premise that the nurse–patient relationship is based on trust, then in order to develop an ethical framework for decision-making, we must also include knowledge about the meaning of respect, privacy, dignity and autonomy from the patient's perspective.

The findings indicate that autonomy is transactional. Taking over the patient's self-choice in daily care may lead to situations where patients accept all decisions made on their behalf. This point of view can even be stretched to include field research; that which is conducted on behalf of patients but does not include them.

Strauss *et al.* (1981) found in a study of psychiatric ideologies and institutions that moral issues became more apparent in the complaints of patients. If the researcher is attuned to patients' situations, then by carefully listening to patients' protests in all types of contexts, knowledge about the interactional basis of moral conflicts can be expanded. One conclusion drawn from this study is that ethical issues in psychiatric nursing most often revolve around the patient who lacks insight, motivation or because of other circumstances, is not capable of self-choice. Moreover, these findings show that a central conflict stems from the nurses' perceived responsibility to limit patients' self-choice on the one hand and to maintain trust on the other.

Communicating Trustworthy Research Results

Compared to conventional research methods, the statistical tests of validity and reliability cannot be applied in field research. Thus, the most important criteria for establishing credibility or trustworthiness of analysis is prolonged engagement, persistent observation and comparison of events (Guba and Lincoln, 1985). This methodological rigour is necessary in order to make the written report, the last phase of the research process, of any scholarly or practical value.

It is therefore important that the written report of qualitative research does not have the appearance of sensational journalism. Since the emergent focus of the study determines the boundaries of inquiry, not all inter-relationships can be fully accounted for in the written report. However, the researcher has an ethical responsibility to carefully describe the methods used and to conduct the analysis so that taking situations *completely* out of their context does not occur. It is essential that the research report contains a discussion on the limitations of the process of inquiry.

An ethical problem with written reports of this kind is that the analysis is based on in-depth interviews. This means that personal identity is known to the researcher and must be kept confidential. The question I posed was, how can this fieldwork be authentically represented and published without divulging information that can lead to breaking confidentiality and, in doing so, harm the persons in the study or even others (e.g. misrepresentation of psychiatric nursing)?

During the process of fieldwork, all observations and interviews that were relevant for the focus of the study were to be coded and categorised. It was therefore important to document the research without losing methodological stringency. In the written report, examples of the main concepts were represented as vignettes in a narrative form. The method of grounded theory itself prevents divulging the personal identity of participants because the aim of the method is to collect and compare incidents and not people. As such, confidentiality of the respondents was maintained. Moreover, all audiotapes of interviews were destroyed after they were transcribed.

It was at this last stage of the research process that I became aware of the problem of having a research advisor who is also chief of staff. While I had deliberately chosen a setting that was unfamiliar in order to counteract bias effects, for the physician who has a responsibility for the management of the ward, bias is difficult to avoid. Moreover, not all of the results portrayed a positive picture of the ward. When published, the study could be criticised for exposing a potentially negative side of psychiatric nursing. This meant that it was necessary to discuss the results not as "truths" but as a result of my interaction with one particular "reality" that is constantly changing and constructed over time. Thus, the findings must be supported by a conscientious description of the whole process of fieldwork. One way was writing the study as a publication for a nursing journal, because it would then be criticised according to the standard reviewing process.

Ethical Considerations for Future Fieldwork

In the following I will list a number of points that I believe are worth considering in future fieldwork.

(1) Even the experienced researcher needs someone with whom to discuss the ethical problems that arise in research. Therefore, it is important that the researcher (novice as well as experienced) doing fieldwork, has access to an adviser who is skilled and experienced in qualitative research.

(2) Conflicts of interest can be avoided by not having the chief of staff (or anyone else in a position of responsibility, or authority over the setting or group to be studied) act as research adviser.

(3) Careful preparation should include discussing with the people to be studied the possibility that certain fieldwork observations might be interpreted as bad practice. Discuss with the staff how to deal with this possibility.

(4) Even if the focus for research is what nurses do, and especially if the study involves participant observation in a long-term care setting, the consent of the patients should be obtained, if at all possible.

Lastly, the ultimate goal of research is theory development, and thus the main question to be asked is: will nursing research of this type contribute to nursing knowledge? In the case of the study described here, the results have led to continued research in ethical decision-making, thus increasing extant knowledge of biomedical ethics. Furthermore, bringing to light the moral aspect of nursing, especially in areas of controversy, also compels us to turn our attention to vulnerable patients. In this way field research in nursing is a necessary moral enterprise.

References

Becker, H. *et al.* (1968) *Boys in White*. Chicago: University of Chicago Press.

Bunch, E.H. (1983) *Everyday Reality of the Psychiatric Nurse. A Study of the Communication Patterns Between the Schizophrenic and the Psychiatric Nurse*. Oslo: Gyldendal Norsk forlag.

Evaneshko, V. (1985) Entrée strategies for nursing filed research studies. In Leininger, M. (ed.) *Qualitative Research Methods in Nursing*. London: Grune and Stratton.

Giorgi, A. (1985) *Phenomenology and Psychological Research*. Pittsburgh: Duquesne University Press.

Glaser, B. and Strauss, A. (1967) *The Discovery of Grounded Theory*. New York: Aldine de Gruyter.

Goffman, E. (1959) *The Presentation of Self in Everyday Life*. Edinburgh: Social Science Research Centre.

Goffman, E. (1961) *Asylums, Essays on the Social Situation of Mental Patients*. New York: Doubleday Anchor.

Lee, R. (1993) *Doing Research on Sensitive Topics*. London, Sage.

Lincoln, Y. and Guba, E. (1985) *Naturalistic Inquiry*. London: Sage.

Lützén, K. (1993) *Moral Sensitivity, A Study of Subjective Aspects of Moral Decision Making in Psychiatric Nursing Practice*. Doctoral Dissertation, Karolinska Institute, Stockholm, Sweden.

Rose, P. and Miller, N. (1986) *The Power of Psychiatry*, Oxford: Polity Press.

Sachs, L. and Krantz, I. (1991) *Anthropology of Medicine and Society*. Stockholm: Repro Print.

Schatzman, L. and Strauss, A. (1973) *Field Research*. Englewood Cliffs, New Jersey: Prentice Hall.

Strauss, A. *et al.* (1981) *Psychiatric Ideologies and Institutions*. London: Transaction Books.

7

Collecting Data from People with Cancer and Their Families: What are the Implications?

Barbara Johnson and Hilary Plant

This chapter sets out some of the ethical and moral issues which emerged during the research process of study designed to investigate peoples' perceptions of need during the first year following a diagnosis of cancer.

The social and emotional toll of coping with cancer has been increasingly recognised and researched over the past 20 years. It is argued that most, if not all, patients affected by cancer are likely to suffer a variety of psychological and social problems in coping with their disease (Williams, 1988). Furthermore, the emotional upheaval produced by the illness itself is often exacerbated by the consequences of aggressive treatment and adjuvant therapy (Bruish and Lyles, 1981). The lives of the family and friends of these patients are also unavoidably linked with such suffering (Northouse, 1984; Hinds, 1992; Sales, 1992).

However, there seems to be little agreement about which methods of research are most appropriately applied to this complex and sensitive area. Much of the emphasis has been on creating instruments to measure the level of distress experienced by patients (Maguire, 1976; Maguire *et al.*, 1978, 1980; Greer, 1988; Slevin, 1992). Whilst most of the research has been undertaken in hospital and in clinical settings it has tended to concentrate on diagnosis, the crisis points and the terminal phase of the illness. Little research has explored what life outside hospitals and clinics is really like for people with cancer and their families who live with the knowledge of a cancer diagnosis and its subsequent management.

In the present study we planned to do a piece of qualitative research which would look at people's perception of need based on their personal experience of cancer. We believed that there may be a mismatch between what patients and their families felt they needed in terms of help and support and what professional carers believed they required. Thus we designed a study which involved interviewing people in their own home on three occasions during the first 13 months following a diagnosis of cancer. We did not want to take a single "snapshot picture" of their experiences but rather we hoped to find out how people's experience of living with a diagnosis of cancer might change with time. We wanted to find out what life was like for patients and their families whilst living away from the professional support offered by hospitals and clinics.

Our interest in exploring the needs of people confronted with a life threatening disease stemmed from our nursing background and our experience in providing information and support for people with cancer and their families. At the outset we saw our research role as impassive, neutral and non-judgemental. We were not there to create an impression or change anything; indeed it was our aim not to. However, the emotional, professional and moral unease that ensued from this decision meant that initially we were constantly trying to cheat the research design until we settled to a more comfortable agreement to "be ourselves" during the research process.

Study Design

Some time was spent in considering carefully the design of the study in order to avoid as far as possible inadvertent distress to participants. Consultants from seven health districts were invited to refer to the project patients newly diagnosed with one of the more common cancers, i.e. breast, colo-rectum, prostate, skin and lung. They were not required to explain the study to participants but were asked to fill in a consent form detailing the words they had used when explaining the diagnosis of cancer to the patient. For example, some patients were told they had "a lump" or "active cells" or simply that they had "cancer". At this stage consultants were merely consenting to our contacting their patients and not seeking the patient's consent for interview. We presumed that the consultant responsible for completing the consent form relied upon either their memory or the patient's notes when recording what a patient had been told about their diagnosis.

Central to our enquiry was the fact that participants were aware of their diagnosis and were able to disclose it to the researcher. Information about treatment or prognosis was not sought as such information was not necessary for the purpose of recruitment. General practitioners were also advised of our intention to invite their patients to participate in the study. This provided them with an opportunity of letting us know if, for whatever reason, they felt approaching a particular patient was inappropriate.

People referred to the study as potential participants were contacted initially by a letter which briefly explained the study using the words recorded on the consultant's consent form. The letter offered participants an early opportunity to refuse further contact with the researcher. Unless we heard to the contrary, the letter was followed approximately a week later by a telephone call from the researcher. If they agreed, participants were then visited at home (or venue of their choice). One of our aims in conducting the research in the home environment was to encourage people to perhaps speak more freely without the fear of jeopardising their treatment or offending the professionals caring for them. During the initial home visit, following a careful explanation of the study and a guarantee *vis-à-vis* confidentiality, participants were asked if they would consent to take part in the project.

The interview took place at the time of the initial visit or a few days later, depending on how the participant felt about the timing of the interview. In essence, they were invited to give an account of what had happened to them from the time they first thought something was wrong (in terms of their health) to the time of the interview.

The second and third interviews at approximately seven and 13 months, however, were somewhat more focused in that participants were asked to give accounts of incidents, both "good" and "bad", that had been of particular significance to them during the time they had been coping with a diagnosis of cancer. Referred to as the "critical incident technique" (Flanagan, 1954; Bliss and Ogborn, 1977, 1987), the method avoids generalities and focuses on actual events and the reasons for their importance.

A small number of "patient" participants were asked at the end of their first interview to identify the person whom they felt had been most affected by their illness. They were then asked if they agreed to the researcher approaching this person to take part in a study looking at the experiences of those close to someone with cancer. The relatives who consented to take part were also interviewed on three occasions. In these interviews a grounded theory approach (Glaser and Strauss, 1967) was used where, instead of eliciting critical incidents, the interview focused more on issues arising from data previously collected. If the patient died during the study, a bereavement interview was carried out several months later with those relatives willing to participate.

A questionnaire was completed at the end of each interview asking the participants for demographic information and details of their contact with health professionals since the time of discharge from hospital. It also included a question about how they, as participants in the study, might be feeling having completed the interview. We believed that completing a questionnaire of this kind would also be an effective way of debriefing participants before finally leaving their home. Participants were also offered a general information leaflet listing addresses and telephone numbers of the various cancer organisations.

Interviews were tape-recorded and transcribed verbatim. To protect their confidentiality participants were given a pseudonym and serial number and, during transcription, no health professional, hospital or clinic was referred to by name.

Participants' perceptions of need were to be identified by examining the accounts of their experiences when affected by cancer. Thus the study design included the assumption that participants had acknowledged their diagnosis and required them to recall and discuss their personal experiences in considerable depth.

Sample

A sample of people (135), believed to have been informed of a cancer diagnosis, and a small sample of their families and friends (28) were referred to the study. Of these, 121 patients and 26 relatives agreed to be interviewed. A small number of patients were not approached by the researcher either because they failed to meet the criteria for inclusion (four), their general practitioner felt it was inappropriate for them to participate (two), they were too ill (one) or they had died (two). Fourteen people did not want to participate because in general they did not want to relive the events of recent months. Of the participants interviewed at least once, a small number withdrew from the study (15) because they felt that they had "put it all behind" them and "couldn't go through it again" (four), had recurrent disease and were too poorly (one) or had died (10).

The research was conducted over a wide geographical area and involved interviewing people aged between 18 and 75 years from a variety of social backgrounds. Apart from our initial telephone call, we (the researchers) had not met any of the participants prior to arriving on their doorstep with the intention of introducing ourselves and the study as well as securing an interview that same day.

Issues Arising from the Study

For reasons of presentation, the issues arising during the study are discussed under three headings:

- accessing participants and gaining consent;
- impact of the interview on the participant and researcher;
- role of the researcher.

However, as will emerge, they do not fall neatly into categories and therefore they overlap to some degree.

Accessing participants and gaining consent

Very early in the project we encountered problems with assessing and gaining consent which forced us to change the study design in order to be able to continue with the research. In referring participants to the study, consultants were asked to state what patients had been told about their diagnosis. Implicit in this approach was the assumption that participants had acknowledged their diagnosis and would be happy to disclose the same to the researcher. Therefore gaining their consent for participation in the study involved assent that they had been given a diagnosis of cancer.

Early problems

During the early interviews it became evident that no assumptions could be safely made about patients' acknowledgement of their diagnosis. This led to difficulties in being able to disclose the true nature of the research to a number of participants and the following are just a few examples of how some reacted to the initial disclosure of the line of enquiry.

First, the participant may never have been told their diagnosis but instead had construed that they had cancer. For example,

> Well . . . nobody actually told me I had cancer . . . I just assumed it was cancer . . . I could just tell . . . but nobody has actually told me . . .

The issue here is that the researcher may then advertently or inadvertently confirm the diagnosis to the participant. The full impact of such disclosure may elude the researcher at the time of interview but may be raised and discussed by the participant at a subsequent interview:

> It didn't hit me at the time . . . but I realised afterwards that I'd had cancer . . . it was just that nobody had actually used the word until you did . . . the last time . . .

Alternatively the referring consultant in a written statement may have notified the researcher of what was believed to have been explained to the participants at the time of the diagnosis. However, the participant may not have internalised the information and therefore did not acknowledge the same reported diagnosis to the researcher, a phenomenon often referred to in the literature as "denial" (Greer, 1988). An example of this was where the participant who, in spite of being encouraged to explain why he had been in hospital, did not acknowledge his diagnosis to the researcher. Following the interview, the patient's daughter explained to the researcher that on being told by the doctor he had cancer, her father had collapsed. This kind of situation not only left us feeling unable to disclose the nature of our enquiry but also feeling we had been "dishonest" with the participant.

In other instances, the diagnosis was simply not acknowledged in categorical terms to the researcher. It is possible that the participant felt unable to cope with the reactions of others when talking about their cancer diagnosis and therefore they may have actively decided against discussing it with anyone, including the researcher. For example,

> Well it was only a wart apparently . . . but they took it off and I'm fine now . . . everything's fine now . . . so what was it you wanted to know?

Again we felt unable to disclose the true nature of our enquiry which left us feeling very uneasy.

There were also occasions where the participant, informed of their diagnosis, had not disclosed the information to their partner or family. This created difficulties, especially when relatives inadvertently read project correspondence which referred to the diagnosis or when they decided to "sit in" on the interview. In one instance the researcher was negotiating a home visit with a participant when the participant's daughter intervened and asked how it was the researcher knew her father's diagnosis before he (the patient) had been informed? She continued by threatening litigation and a confrontation with the consultant. Later, the consultant confirmed that the patient had been clearly told his diagnosis but had chosen not to disclose it to either his wife or daughter.

There may also be confusion about the words health professionals choose to use when referring to a cancer diagnosis. For example, one woman understood her consultant to have told her she had breast cancer, but when our letter arrived asking her to take part in a study of people with "malignant disease" (the words used by the consultant in his letter of referral) she construed that the disease must have spread through her body. Needless to say our letter caused her much unnecessary pain and anguish until it was realised by her family doctor that she was confusing "malignant" disease with "metastatic" disease.

How then can we, the researchers, explain the nature of our enquiry when there is a very real risk that the participant either does not know their diagnosis or, for some reason, they choose not to disclose it to the interviewer? In the present study we decided to attempt to resolve some of these problems by not disclosing immediately the true line of our enquiry in the letter of introduction we sent to participants. Instead, we waited to explain the purpose of the study until they had acknowledged their diagnosis to us either over the telephone or during the initial visit. We did this by asking them to talk about their recent time in hospital (why they were admitted to hospital; what they understood had been done to them and why, and so on) before explaining the nature of the study and seeking their consent to be interviewed.

Consent

In this kind of research there is a very real problem concerning the ethics of "informed consent". As well as our initial difficulty in discussing the diagnosis there were two further problems in gaining informed consent from our participants. The first of these problems has been addressed by several authors and concerns the difficulty of fully informing the participants of the potential risks and benefits of taking part in research. This is difficult when at the outset the flexible nature of the research means one is unable to predict exactly what the participant is going to say and therefore to know in advance what effect this process may have on them (Larossa *et al.*, 1981; Ramos, 1989; Holloway, 1992;). The concept of qualitative research may be quite difficult for participants to understand and thus hard to prepare them for the possible outcomes. We attempted to deal with this by carefully negotiating each interview, explaining in detail what the participants would be expected to do and emphasising that they could discontinue and withdraw from the interview at any time. Furthermore, as mentioned earlier, the impact of the interview was discussed with each participant after the main body of the interview during the post-interview questionnaire. This will be discussed further under the section dealing with the role of researcher.

We also endeavoured to avoid some of the problems concerning informed consent as detailed by Smith (1992). For example, Smith cautions against delegation of research interviews to inexperienced researchers and any kind of manipulation in order to gain consent to participate. An example of this manipulation is the possibility that some people participate in research studies because they believe that this will benefit their medical care (Smith, 1992). We had believed that because we came from a university rather than a hospital, and because from the outset of the research process we were at pains to distance ourselves from medical care, we would be exempt from this. However, the introductory letter to the patients mentioned their hospital consultant's name, and participants having once made this connection may have felt too vulnerable to refuse our first request to visit them at home, in order to introduce the study.

As the conventional image of the researcher is someone who "neutralises his or her 'irrelevant' identities and viewpoints while conducting research" (Kleinman and Copp, 1993), initially we were uncertain as to whether or not we should disclose our identity as nurses. But in the course of time we decided we would disclose our professional identity where it seemed appropriate. However, we were only too aware that this may also have made it more difficult for people to refuse to participate. Thus in spite of our efforts to make it easy for people to refuse to take part, we realise that, as pointed out by Stacey (1988), in practice it must have been very difficult for participants to "send us away" once we had made the effort to turn up on their doorstep. For example,

I wasn't sure I really wanted to do it [the interview] but when you said on the 'phone that you just wanted to discuss the interview with me I thought "OK then" . . . but then when you came . . . you'd made all that effort . . . I thought I'd better do it . . .

When negotiating access there was also the problem of ascertaining and respecting the participant's level of adjustment to their diagnosis. In the design of the present study we aimed to be sensitive to the participant's level of adjustment, but implicit in asking them to participate was possibly the suggestion that their diagnosis was more serious than they had previously believed it to be. For example, one woman who had been treated for colo-rectal cancer expressed concern about her attitude towards her cancer diagnosis:

I don't think I am taking this seriously enough . . . the cancer I mean . . . I mean to be invited to do this [take part in the study] must mean it's a bit serious . . .

On the other hand one man presumed that he had been invited to participate because he had made such a remarkable recovery from his surgery, although in reality we were aware that his long term prognosis was uncertain.

Impact of the interview on the participant

Little is known about the effect a research interview may have on a participant. The design of our study required participants to reflect, recall and recount their experiences from the time they first thought something was wrong to the time of the interview. It is perhaps worth noting that at the time of the first interview many participants described themselves as "disease free" by remarking that they "no longer had cancer" and "had put it all behind them now". Other participants, particularly those with lung and colo-rectal cancer were aware they were not disease free and may die from their illness. Thus is was from these different positions that participants tried to tell their story.

Some attempts have been made by researchers to follow up the impact on participants immediately following an interview (Eardley *et al.*, 1991). In the present study we tried to do this by asking participants, at the end of each interview, to describe how they were feeling having recalled their experiences over recent months. We realise that such an approach was possibly biased in that participants might be unwilling to be too honest with a researcher who has just spent two or more hours interviewing them! Furthermore, they may not have been fully aware of the long- and-short term effects of participation at the time of interview. The danger for us as researchers was the implicit assumption that participants might find it beneficial to talk about their experiences and more especially to someone who has time and space to listen. However, in the present study, we did occasionally find the contrary to be true.

Costs and benefits of the interview to the participant

From our experience the kind of interview process in which we engaged conferred both costs and benefits on participants. However, as mentioned previously, it was impossible to clarify these for the participant prior to interview. We will discuss "costs" and "benefits" under the same heading because, in our experience, what appeared to be a cost to one participant was of benefit to another. For example,

> I found that talking about things was really helpful . . . I haven't been able to talk like this to anyone . . .

and

> I thought that talking about things would be OK . . . I mean I'm doing a counselling course at the moment so it has to be OK doesn't it? But actually you know I am not so sure about all this business of letting it all hang out . . . I'm not sure at all . . . I found it all very distressing . . .

Thus it is very difficult to judge what may be of "cost" and what may be of "benefit" to a particular individual. Different participants have different experiences and assess these experiences in different ways, which of course may alter with the passage of time. For example.

> Well I felt OK at the time . . . I thought it was good to talk about things . . . it helped me to understand things a bit better . . . but then that night I felt dreadful . . . I cried most of the night . . . my husband was very worried . . . it had brought it all back to me . . . but now I feel OK again . . . perhaps it was just one of those things . . . you don't want me to go over all that again do you?

Then there were those who worried about being upset by the interview. For those who had "put the thing behind" them, reliving and recounting their so-called cancer experience became a difficult decision for them to make. In such instances it also became difficult for the researcher to know "what line to take" next. No guarantees or reassurances could be offered and therefore the participant was often left unaided to make the decision for themselves. However, in the majority of cases the participant confirmed later how much the interview had helped them. But what about those who had not been helped?

Potential costs

Being informed. In this instance the participants may learn or be told something by the researcher they would otherwise have preferred not to know. For example, as previously discussed they may be given, albeit inadvertently, confirmation of their diagnosis.

Being reminded. For many participants the interview serves to remind them of events which, as part of this coping strategy, they may have chosen to put to "the back of their minds". For example,

> Each time you come it reminds me how serious it really is. I do try and push it to the back of my mind.

Being disturbed. Some participants reported at the end of the interview that they had found the experience of reliving events very disturbing. For example, one participant, a man who had been treated for cancer of the prostate said that old feelings had been "churned up" – feelings that he had long since forgotten about.

On the other hand, a few participants reported at the following interview that they had felt very disturbed after the previous interview. Such feelings were often only manifest some time after the interview, for example the following day. One woman described herself as feeling fine immediately after the interview, but at the subsequent interview some weeks later she told the researcher:

> I thought I was alright after the interview but that evening I felt very depressed . . . somehow it all came back to me . . . my husband was a bit annoyed . . . it went on for several days . . . I'd decided I wouldn't do the next interview . . .

Being threatened. For a few participants, recounting events raised doubts in their minds about the current status of their cancer. Many talked about the cancer having "gone", although many were aware that the cancer could "come back" or recur at any time in the future. Nevertheless, going back over events seemed to raise doubts in their minds.

Potential benefits

For the majority of people the experience of the interview was considered "helpful" and in some instances even cathartic. Many participants described it as the first opportunity they had had to talk about wh had happened to them and how they had felt about it at the time. Some felt anxious talking "about cancer" to their family and friends but welcomed the opportunity to talk to an outsider. For example,

> It's actually the first time I've talked to anyone . . . I cried the last two times and I think it does you good. Afterwards you feel better that you've let the emotion out because somewhere that's been bottled up . . . I think . . . you need to do it.

By expressing and releasing feelings, often by crying or showing anger, some participants felt that being interviewed had benefited them. At a less intense level some participants found the interview simply "helpful" or that it helped them to order their thoughts and feelings. For example,

> I honestly think it has been very therapeutic . . . I think it has done me a lot of

good. You didn't counsel me . . . you just let me talk. I didn't want to talk about it . . . I just wanted to bury it . . . but it has brought it out . . . my thoughts . . . my feelings . . . which is very good . . .

There could be several reasons why participants felt they had benefited from taking part in the study. The above quote suggests that the interview was cathartic because it allowed people to express themselves freely and voice their fears without the fear of being judged or advised how to cope with their feelings.

For some participants the notion of helping others "who might follow" was also considered a positive outcome of participation. As Reisman (1976) argues, when people believe they are talking about themselves in order to help someone else, that is the "helper-therapy principle", participation can be of considerable benefit to the participant.

That the research was beneficial was by far the most common response by participants to the interview. Following our first meeting, we were usually greeted warmly and with great hospitality on our return visits. Indeed, on a number of occasions, participants insisted on showing their appreciation by producing a hand-made gift or produce from the garden. Many expressed great enthusiasm about the purpose of the research and were careful to remember what had happened in the interim. For some, particularly the relatives, it seemed to validate their experience.

There were a number of potential drawbacks, however, even when the research did appear to confer benefits. There was no therapeutic contract with the participant. The contract was simply to collect data and offer an information leaflet to the participant at the end of the interview. Thus, although encouraging participants to talk frankly and openly about their experiences following a cancer diagnosis may have afforded some temporary relief, something might be started which then might remain unfinished. In other words, offering an outlet and then withdrawing it could potentially be quite harmful to participants (Larossa *et al.*, 1981; de Raeve, 1992).

Some possible solutions

There were several steps we took to reduce the potential "costs" of the interview to participants. First, during the entire interview we attempted to respect the participant's level of adjustment to their cancer diagnosis. Second, we permitted the interview to run its full course whenever possible so that participants would be able to complete what they wanted to say and not be left with unfinished business. Thus we ran contrary to the more conventional research interview practice where the recommendation is to try and keep within a time limit. Third, as discussed earlier, we tried to debrief the particip-ant at the end of each interview and gave them the project secretary's telephone number as well as our personal number, should they have wanted to "tell us any more" or have felt the need to "talk to someone". Fourth, in the event of being very concerned about a participant's well-being, we discussed with them the possibility of referring them to an appropriate professional. Because such action entailed a breachf confidentiality, it was only taken in those circumstances where the participant agreed to being referred by ourselves. Such provision was not planned for, but during the early stages of the project we learned that it was important to deal with our concerns at the time of the interview rather than going home and later worrying about it.

Our personal interventions into these sometimes difficult situations will be described later under the heading of the role of the researcher.

Impact of the interview on the researcher

During the study the concerns arising for the researcher ranged from gaining ethical approval, data collection, disengagement, data handling and data representation. Ethical approval was granted on the condition that participants would not be caused any further and unnecessary anxiety or stress beyond that with which they were already coping. However, as researchers we could only offer assurances that every effort would be made not to "upset" the participant and clearly the ambiguity of such a condition, when some people did indeed get upset during their interview, left us questioning the terms on which ethical approval had been granted.

Accessing participants on their territory can be threatening both for the researcher and the researched, particularly for the untrained and inexperienced home visitor. In the early stages of the study, anxiety was often generated by the uncertainty of our role whilst trying to access data. We often jokingly referred to this as the "blind date" (Ball, 1990). In other words, to what extent did we have to "play the game" in order to get a participant's consent to interview?

In addition to the concerns we experienced in respect of accessing and collecting data, there were problems associated with the more practical aspects of the study. Fieldwork was often undertaken some considerable distance from both the research institution and the researchers' homes. Furthermore, to accommodate participants, some interviews had to be undertaken during the evening or at the weekend. This situation often led to the researcher feeling isolated and unsupported for several days or even weeks, at a time. We felt that there were inherent risks in working alone and that being able to return to "base camp" most days would be in the interest of both the research and the researcher.

There were other concerns arising from carrying out fieldwork in people's homes. Travelling to and from interviews was costly in terms of both time and energy. For example,

1.30am. I've had a very difficult evening. Not only is the weather appalling (very foggy and icy) but it's taken me two hours to get home and the car is playing up . . . I got lost in the fog on the way home . . . I am worried about Jane [participant] and I need to talk with someone about this . . . but my family has gone to bed . . . and I want to go too . . . (field notes).

The length of interviews varied. We realised early in the study that arranging an interview in the afternoon to follow a morning interview could present difficulties for both the researcher and the participant. For a number of unforeseeable reasons the morning interview may be protracted and in addition, conducting two successive interviews proved to be physically and emotionally overtaxing for the researcher. Another problem arising from the lengthy interviews was the process of disengagement. This was sometimes very difficult especially if the person lived alone or if they had prepared food and anticipated we would stay and share it with them. After one or two difficult experiences of this nature, we agreed we would be prepared to accept any offer of hospitality. In some instances the problem of disengagement continued long after the project had been completed and to this day both of us still have contact with one or two participants.

Listening to people's stories (told for the benefit of our research) at times had a tremendous and powerful impact on both of us. The stories were sometimes very emotionally charged and we often felt that we were left to absorb such emotion without the "protection" or "distraction" of professional role and institution. The difficulties we encountered during fieldwork were compounded by our feelings of loneliness and isolation. One or two mentors suggested that some of our concerns stemmed directly from a lack of control over the research process, a reaction reported elsewhere in the literature (Kleinman and Copp, 1993). Thus for a while we were left believing that our concerns merely reflected some kind of shortcoming in ourselves as fieldworkers. However, we became aware that colleagues working in similar areas of research were also experiencing similar problems but there was no forum to discuss and reason with this particular aspect of the research process. In a bid to help ourselves, a small group of us (six researchers) met fortnightly in a support group with a college psychotherapist as facilitator to discuss our concerns arising from the fieldwork and the effect they were having on the research process and our wellbeing.

The role of researchers in data collection

During the fieldwork our initial intention was to minimise the potential ripple effect on participants' lives, whilst at the same time trying to capture a picture of their experiences which did not interfere with their medical position (about which we knew very little). We planned our role as the conventional positivist researcher (Denzin, 1989). However, in a short time this approach created an impossible conflict for us and as mentioned earlier we found ourselves cheating our own rules constantly. In time we became very influenced by and relieved to learn from both the feminist and ethnographic literature that our conflict and difficulties were shared by others (Oakley, 1981; Cannon, 1989; Ball, 1990). Thus we endeavoured to make the interview a more reciprocal encounter for both researcher and participant. We resolved to enable participants to have more control over their interview. This we did by offering them control of the tape recorder and copies of their transcripts if they wanted them. We decided that if we felt concerned about a participant we would answer questions raised by them and disclose our identity as nurses. We also became aware that the nature of our interview encouraged participants to develop the kind of relationship which is founded on trust and which invariably involved them in who and what we are beyond that of interviewer. However, we then developed a further concern. As Stacey (1988) argues, by giving more of ourselves to the participants and thus engaging them more actively in the study, we were making it more difficult for them to refuse to participate if they so wished.

We are left with some concerns which we have found impossible to resolve. As researchers we felt uncomfortable if, for example, the participants related instances of bad professional practice. It was even more difficult if we recognised a problem with care or treatment and they did not. Some examples of this include where a participant had not been informed of their diagnosis yet clearly wanted to be informed; where a participant appeared to have been misinformed of their diagnosis and/or treatment and where a participant disclosed something disturbing, for example threatening to commit suicide or failing to comply with medical treatment. Furthermore, our promise of confidentiality became a problem. Because of our contract with the participant, that is, "Anything you say to me will remain between you, me and transcriber", we at times became burdened with information which we felt we wanted to (and indeed believed we should) discuss with their carers and others.

We discussed earlier how, when concerned about issues of confidentiality, we resolved that we would deal with the concern at the time and ask if we could refer the matter to an appropriate professional carer. However, if the participant did not agree, or if they did not perceive there was a problem and it seemed inappropriate to seek their permission to refer them to another worker or agency, we were left with considerable feelings of disquiet. Not being able to do anything was at times very difficult to live with.

Thus the ethical dilemmas which confronted us became of much greater issue than aspects of the research process (such as data "contamination") which we were committed to initially. To this end, whilst each interview was approached from a common perspective, ultimately each interview became an individual entity. To cause as little harm as possible to the participant and to square with their perceptions of their clinical management and role of their health carers, we adapted our role as researcher during each interview.

However, there remain certain aspects of our experience about which we still feel uneasy. It is possible that a different approach to the research may have pre-empted or resolved some of the outstanding concerns. We believe that addressing issues as they arose and trying to find ways of resolving them moved us forward, both in respect of the study and of our professional skills. Nevertheless, one of our principal recommendations would be that "real time" is planned and budgeted for in a study of this nature. In this way the members of the research team, particularly the fieldworkers, will feel encouraged to raise, explore and hopefully resolve issues as they arise and not feel guilty about spending project time supporting each other.

Acknowledgement

We wish to express gratitude to Cancer Relief Macmillan Fund who funded the project and Dr Alan Cribb, King's College London.

References

Ball, S. (1990) Self-doubt and soft data: social and technical trajectories in ethnographic field work. *Qualitative Studies in Education*, 3(2), 157–171.

Bliss, J. and Ogborn, J. (1977) *Students' Reactions to Undergraduate Science.* Published for the Nuffield Foundation by Heinemann Educational Books, London.

Bliss, J. and Ogborn, J. (1987) Knowledge elicitation. In Ennals J.R. (ed.) *Artificial Intelligence State of the Art Report 15:3.* Oxford: Pergamon Infotech.

Bruish, T. and Lyles, J. (1981) Effectiveness of relaxation training in reducing adverse reactions to cancer chemotherapy. *Journal of Behavioural Medicine*, 4, 65–78.

Cannon, S. (1989) Social research in stressful settings: difficulties for the sociologist studying the treatment of breast cancer. *Sociology of Health and Illness*, 11(1), 66–77.

Denzin, N.K. (1989) *The Research Act.* Englewood Cliffs, NJ: Prentice-Hall.

de Raeve, L. (1992) Ethical issues in palliative nursing research. A question of kind? A question of degree? In *Proceedings of the Seventh International Cancer Nursing Conference, Vienna.* Oxford: Rapid Communications.

Eardley, A., Cribb, A. and Pendleton, L. (1991) Ethical issues in psychosocial research among patients with cancer: a review. *European Journal of Cancer*, 27(2), 166–169.

Flanagan, J.C. (1954) The critical incident technique. *Psychological Bulletin*, **51** (July), 327–358.

Glaser, B. and Strauss, A. (1967) *The Discovery of Grounded Theory*. Chicago: Aldine.

Greer, S. (1988) Measuring mental adjustment to cancer. In M. Watson, S. Greer and C. Thomas (eds) *Psychosocial Oncology*, pp. 45–51. Oxford: Pergamon Press.

Hinds, C. (1992) Suffering: a relatively unexplored phenomenon among family caregivers of non-institutionalised patients with cancer. *Journal of Advanced Nursing*, **17**, 918–925.

Holloway, I. (1992) Patients as participants in research. *Senior Nurse*, **12**(3), 46–47.

Kleinman, S. and Copp, M.A. (1993) *Emotions and Fieldwork*. Sage Publications.

Larossa, R., Bennett, L.A. and Gelles, R.J. (1981) Ethical dilemmas in qualitative family research. *Journal of Marriage and the Family*, May, 303–313.

Maguire, G.P. (1976) The psychiatric and social sequelae of mastectomy. In Howells J.G. (ed.) *Modern Perspectives in the Psychiatric Aspects of Surgery*, pp. 390–420. New York: Brunner Mazel.

Maguire, G.P., Lee, E.G., Bevington, D.J., Kuchemann, C.S., Crabtree, R.J. and Cornell, C.E. (1978) Psychiatric problems in the first year after mastectomy. *British Medical Journal*, **1**, 963–965.

Maguire, G.P., Tait, A., Brooke, M., Thomas, C., Howat, J.M.T., Sellwood, R.A. and Bush, H. (1980) Psychiatric morbidity and physical toxicity associated with adjuvant chemotherapy after mastectomy. *British Medical Journal*, **281**, 1179–1180.

Northouse, L. (1984) The impact of cancer on the family: an overview. *International Journal of Psychiatry in Medicine*, **14**(3), 215–242.

Oakley, A. (1981) Interviewing women: a contradiction in terms. In Roberts, H. (ed.) *Doing Feminist Research*. Routledge & Kegan Paul, London.

Ramos, M.C. (1989) Some ethical issues of qualitative research. *Research in Nursing and Health*, **12**, 57–63.

Reisman, F. (1976) How does self help work? *Social Policy*, **7**(2), 41–45.

Sales, E. (1992) Psychosocial impact of the phase of cancer on the family: an updated review. *Journal of Psychosocial Oncology*, **9**(4), 1–18.

Slevin, M.L. (1992) Quality of life: philosophical question or clinical reality? *British Medical Journal*, **305**, 466–469.

Smith, L. (1992) Ethical issues in interviewing. *Journal of Advanced Nursing*, **17**, 98–103.

Stacey, J. (1988) Can there be a feminist ethnography? *Women's Studies International Forum*, **11**(1), 21–27.

Williams, C. (1988) Psychological consequences of the diagnosis and management of cancer: a physician's view. In M. Watson, S. Greer and C. Thomas (eds) *Psychosocial Oncology*, pp. 119–126. Oxford: Pergamon Press.

II

Three Perspectives

8

Ethical Commentary

Louise de Raeve

The preceding seven chapters have described a series of ethical issues, dilemmas and reactions experienced by nurse researchers. It is now my intention to draw some comparisons and contrasts between these chapters and in so doing, I shall try to do justice to the complexity and richness of the descriptions presented. My analysis will be grouped under the following headings:

1. *Rationale*, i.e. why do this piece of research?
2. *Methodology*, i.e. why this approach rather than that and what can be said to be the particular moral issues that arise from using a certain methodology?
3. *Access* including consent and the function of gatekeepers. This chapter will not, however, address the question of ethical review by committee as Chapter 11 is devoted to this.
4. *The role of the researcher*, with particular attention being given to role conflict and role ambiguity.
5. *The benefits and harms* of the research from the participants' point of view.
6. *Publication and Confidentiality*.
7. *Termination*.

On a careful reading of the preceding chapters, I noticed that many writers refer to the idea of deception, but without always making it quite clear exactly what they have in mind. Similarly, a distinction between anonymity and confidentiality is referred to without any very clear analysis of what this might mean. These issues will be examined in the following discussion.

Rationale

As Roger Watson (Chapter 1) remarks, "It could be considered unethical to proceed with any kind of research involving patients, if the researcher is not absolutely certain why the research is being carried out" and this of course includes satisfying oneself "that the information which is being sought is not available elsewhere" (Watson, p. 8). Thus the mere need to do a research project for one's degree would not be a morally adequate justification, in isolation, for embarking on research. Jill Rogers (Chapter 2) introduces the idea that in this planning stage, information about other similar studies may assist one in designing one's own study in order not to repeat mistakes or so that one can produce data that can be meaningfully compared with data gathered in previous research. "It was therefore possible to draw on some of the methodology from this study and to pursue some similar issues" (Rogers, p. 21).

Methodology

Rationale of course connects with issues of methodology, since it is both a pragmatic and a moral matter that the tools, i.e. the method, should be suitable for doing the job. Clearly, one should be using the method best suited to obtaining the results sought. Not to do so threatens to produce invalid and inconsequential data and to have wasted a lot of people's time. In addition, participants might have good grounds for feeling deceived, since their co-operation would presumably have been sought on the basis that the research was considered to be valuable. This possibility of wasting people's time matters deeply, for many may put themselves out to participate. Consider, for example, the effort the health authorities went to, to facilitate Jill Rogers' work or the emotional effort that people were prepared to make in contributing to Johnson and Plant's study (Chapter 7). Some patients, particularly those with life-threatening illnesses may have little time left, so it had better be good research to justify using it.

Under the sections on consent and benefits and harms, more detailed comments will be made concerning the specific ethical features of some of the methodologies used. However, it is worth noting the extent to which, in the preceding chapters, the bias is towards methodologies from the social sciences which rely on techniques such as participant observation and unstructured or semi-structured interviews, with a tendency towards the production of qualitative rather than quantitative data. The lack of comprehension about these methods in the medical-scientific community is a familiar protest amongst nurses and social scientists, as Lathlean (Chapter 3, p. 34) describes.

In Chapter 10, I shall examine some issues of method more fully. One feature, however, which may compound misunderstanding is that these different methodologies tend to use the same words to capture very different concepts, e.g. "sample" and "validity". Ethical review might be a smoother process for nursing research if the language used reflected the differences of various approaches rather than introducing apparent similarity. The latter may serve to simply exasperate those who have a bias towards types of research where such words have considerable precision of meaning. Other words do exist in the literature, for example Heron talks about "coherence" (Heron, 1988, p. 43) as being his understanding of "validity" in the context of his research approach. It might save a lot of misunderstanding to use the language that fits precisely. "Validity" is rather a "catch-all" concept, conveying something general to do with the trustworthiness of results but its exact meaning seems tied to specific research contexts.

Access

Some truly fascinating issues are raised here, and one has to pay tribute to the researchers in their attempts to negotiate this minefield with sensitivity and to thank them for their honest admission of wisdom sometimes achieved with painful hindsight.

One of the central questions that arises is the issue of how "neutral" is participant observation when conducted in an environment where normally private experiences (being in bed etc.) are conducted in a public/semi-public place (a ward). "Intrusion can be seen in terms of being an observer in areas which would otherwise be private, which may be problematic in sensitive settings such as hospitals" (Ersser, Chapter 4, p. 48). Even in ordinary public settings, staring is considered rude or offensive and children are taught not to do it. Only in contexts of shared intimacy does prolonged looking acquire the acceptability of "gazing".

In Sylvia Buckingham's study (Chapter 5, p. 66), one wonders what the mother might have made of this nurse contriving to be near the cubicle and peeping in at intervals. It might have passed unnoticed but possibly not. Is it legitimate to be observing other people's children for purposes that parents are unaware of, regardless of how much it is or is not judged to be in the child's potential interests to do so? An interesting comparison could perhaps be made with schools. Parents might tolerate the presence of a trainee teacher as an observer in the classroom but they might protest at the presence of a researcher, unless their prior permission had been sought.

It is Kim Lützén (Chapter 6, p. 83) who raises the question of the consent of parties within the field of vision, even if they are not specifically the focus of the study, and she describes how, inevitably, patients made contact with her (Lützén, p. 81). This of course introduces the interesting question of power since patients are not usually considered to be in charge of the ward territory in which they may happen to live for considerable periods of time. Lützén usefully points out that the researcher may unwittingly step into and perpetuate power relationships which occur within the institutions which are being studied. This theme of power is further explored by Ersser (p. 50), Rogers (p. 23) and Lathlean (p. 37–38) in terms of how individuals/organisations may perceive approaches via institutional bodies that have power over them and how this may interfere with the capacity of individuals or groups of individuals to give uncoerced voluntary consent.

Johnson and Plant clearly took great pains to inform relevant people, for example GPs, of the nature of the research, but their approach to the actual participants is interesting for its "opt out" rather than "opt in" emphasis. "The letter offered participants an early opportunity to refuse further contact with the researcher. Unless we heard to the contrary, the letter was followed approximately a week later by a telephone call from the researcher" (Johnson and Plant, p. 87). Is this or is it not subtle pressure and even if it is, is it justified? Presumably, researchers would fear that to have an "opt in" requirement would leave one with a very small population to study but unless this is tested it remains fantasy rather than reality. Perhaps one might be surprised.

One cannot escape the researcher's need to accomplish a worthwhile piece of research and hence one can imagine the frustration of not having adequate numbers of participants. Understandable as this may be, however, it is worth reflecting on these words:

> The author found herself changing voice tone and manner when, after several attempts to gain subjects, she had been less successful than planned. In other words, she began to sound more assertive; the value of the work to them and others was emphasized. Participation was actively encouraged by saying how much their help would be appreciated. In all these things, the audience was manipulated in order to achieve the sample (Smith, 1992, p. 100).

Roger Watson (pp. 10–12) raises the interesting question of consent by proxy, and the legal aspect of this is commented upon by Bridgit Dimond in Chapter 9. The issue of proxy consent is frequently referred to in American literature and, in relation to this, UK nurses may need to be careful when extrapolating from such sources. The legislation on consent can be very different between States and between some States and the UK. In focusing on the moral rather than the legal perspective of research with people who are deemed incompetent to consent, it may be very important to consult with a close friend or relative to help determine what could be considered to be in the individual's best interests. In addition, it is likely to help preserve trust between family members and health care professionals and (assuming benevolent intentions) therefore also to be in the elderly person's interests. Advance consent to research (Watson, p. 12), along the lines of an advance directive does not appear to be a promising avenue to pursue, apart from the light it may throw on a best interests assessment. As with all advance statements, the difficulty lies in determining how much a decision made in one state of mind can really be said to apply to situations where circumstances are very different

(Robertson, 1991, p. 7). At best, such directives offer an indication of what the person *might* have wanted to do.

Watson (p. 13) refers to the idea of selective consent being discriminatory: "We felt that to use selective consent in this way would be to discriminate in favour of those patients who were fortunate enough to have residual cognitive skills and privileged enough to have regular visitors." This is a comprehensible point of view, but since it is easily reversible and one could argue that those who could have given their consent but were not consulted were being equally discriminated against, it does not seem a very morally persuasive argument.

Several writers are concerned about consent and deception (Buckingham, p. 62; Watson, p. 7; Ersser, p. 43–46). Watson expresses the view that placebo controlled (or no treatment controlled) randomised trials involve "a measure of deceit towards those taking part. Needless to say, such trials should not take place without the appropriate information being given to those involved, but deceit is operated nevertheless." It is true that in such trials harms may result for people through their being denied what turns out to be a good treatment or through their being damaged by a poor treatment and, in the latter case, with the wisdom of hindsight, participants might well view it as a bonus to have been allocated to the placebo branch. I have difficulty, however, in understanding wherein lies the deceit. If people are clearly informed of the nature of randomisation and of all the possibilities of the trial branches, then provided they have understood and their consent is based on the knowledge that some information will be withheld, is this deception? It would be a very strict world to live in, if keeping something secret always equated with deception. As the person from whom the secret was kept, I am likely to make an accusation of deception where I perceive my interests to have suffered from the information having been withheld but, where I can see the justification for secrecy, I may in fact endorse the practice, despite a wish to know.

Other writers raise the question of deception with regard to participant observation either in terms of the researcher not making it clear to the population being studied exactly what is being investigated (Buckingham, p. 62) or in terms of the researcher possibly exploiting the ambiguity between formal data collecting periods and informal socialising (Ersser, p. 45). Johnson and Plant (p. 89) write of sometimes being "unable to disclose the true nature" of their enquiry because of possible participants not seeming to be aware of the true nature of their diagnosis. This left the researchers feeling "very uneasy".

These are all slightly different shades of a similar picture. As with much psychological research, Sylvia Buckingham could not easily have said she was studying nurses' responses to children in pain, as this would have immediately altered these responses. However, it does raise the question of whether one makes it clear to potential participants that one is withholding some information, explains why and promises to divulge this information on completion of the research. Johnson and Plant's predicament was more complex since in their circumstances revelation could never have been broached without the risk of disturbing and upsetting participants. This particular issue raises the question of whether those people who seemed unaware of their diagnosis should have been proper subjects for the research. However, discovering this state of affairs could not have happened until something of a relationship had already been formed between researcher and participant. It could be argued that to invite people to participate and then to drop them from a research study after they have expressed a willingness to participate is also possibly harmful, and more especially so where one could give no clear reason for doing so. Johnson and Plant elected to interview people who had shown a willingness to participate, even if they did not seem to know their diagnosis, but the data from these interviews was not included in the final analysis. As Johnson and Plant have pointed out in a subsequent communication, the dilemma for them was between dropping from the project those people who had shown a willingness to participate versus deceiving them into believing their data would be used in the final analysis. When embarking on the research, they had never imagined such a difficulty since, according to the referrers, all the patients knew their diagnoses.

Ersser's point (p. 45) about possibly exploiting informal gatherings and thus being rather deceptive raises the interesting question of whether a participant observer can and should be seen to be in "informal" mode amongst the population being studied. It also leads directly to the issue of the research role.

Role

One of the best articles on this subject was written in 1979 by May. She states: "If subjects frequently misperceive the nurse-researcher role, then to whom has the research subject given consent – the nurse or the researcher?" (May, 1979, p. 37). Nurses tend to have a benign public image (why else would they be good at recruiting people into trials for medical research?) which of course introduces the possibility of witting or unwitting exploitation by the nurse-researcher. It seems likely that many of the research projects described bene-fited from having a nurse-researcher doing the work; Judith Lathlean, who is not a nurse, states that she employed a nurse as a research associate "to complement my expertise and background" (Lathlean, p. 33). It could be argued that for some of the more ethnographic approaches, the professional background of the researcher would have quite deliberately shaped both the process and the results of the research. It is difficult to imagine how a non-nurse would have effectively pursued the research conducted by either Ersser or Buckingham, which is not to say that a non-nurse could not research in this field, but probably rather different data would have been gathered and different interpretations offered for it. It is interesting that some researchers deliberately chose to work in a context where they were already known (Buckingham) and others equally deliberately chose not to (Lützén). Rogers (p. 26) deliberately employed "interviewers who had no connection with the participants". The pros and cons of this obviously partly depend on the nature of the research being conducted but clearly, if one is known to research participants in a capacity other than researcher, this may well make for easy access but is likely to compound issues to do with role ambiguity and consent.

Ersser (pp. 45–46) describes dilemmas about what to wear, what to say about oneself, etc., and he evidently operated a clear boundary between those nursing tasks, as a researcher, he thought it legitimate to fulfil (helping a patient to walk to the room for the interview (p. 49)) and those he did not (noting the leaking ileostomy tube but informing another nurse of the problem (p. 52)). Johnson and Plant write of a blurring of their role between that of counsellor and researcher and Buckingham (p. 60) talks about a relationship of friendship and of becoming "one of the team". It is normal for the recipients of friendly understanding and sympathy to become progressively attached to those who make such overtures, and as Johnson and Plant (p. 98) observe, such attitudes may make it increasingly difficult for participants to refuse to participate or to withdraw from the research. Buckingham felt that a sense of connection and familiarity with the nurses she was studying contributed towards making it more difficult to "intercede in situations where I was unhappy about nursing practice" (p. 60). The converse side of this is of course that the more trusting the relationship between researcher and researched, the greater is the researcher's access to deeply personal data.

It is Sylvia Buckingham, I think, who gives the clearest expression to the central dilemma of nurse researchers when she says: "My primary concern was for the child and I decided that I must intervene if no other staff recognised that the child was in pain" (Buckingham, p. 62). No nurse is going to quarrel with this, but of course one needs to see what in practice such an assertion amounted to. Here, one finds that it was a baseline position for when something deeply negligent or dangerous transpired but, for lesser inadequacies of practice, the principle was relinquished in favour of the need to gather data and not to upset relationships, thereby preserving the participants' engagement in the research. Other factors such as time were also relevant, but clearly nurse-researchers need to first examine exactly what their motivations *are*, not what they think they *ought* to be and then debate these matters within the profession. Sally Borbasi (1994) appears to share this concern for greater debate.

It seems that an inevitable feature of most research is that one is prepared to sacrifice, to some extent, the needs of a current population in favour of the imagined or predicted benefits for future populations. As Munhall observes: "Technically, the research enterprise turns people into means [i.e. 'means' to the research 'end'], and though one could argue that this occurs far less with qualitative research, the potential still remains" (Munhall, 1988, p. 155). It is a matter of moral opinion as to whether or not this "trade-off" is justifiable, but, even for those for whom it is, approval is likely to depend on guarantees of restricted contexts and built-in constraints. How such constraints may be institutionalised will be further explored in Chapters 9 and 11, but this still leaves open the self-regulation of professions such as nursing. Codes of research practice (e.g. ; *National Institute for Nursing, 1993; Royal College of Nursing, 1993*) may only be a start.

Many people find it deeply morally troubling to think that others are being used *merely* as a means to any kind of end. History reveals plenty of shocking examples of the lengths that human beings seem prepared to go in their treatment of each other, once arguments suggesting that desirable ends justify the means needed to achieve them gain widespread purchase. It should be remembered, however, that people frequently use each other as a means to an end, for example the use I make of rubbish collectors to empty my dustbin or bus drivers to get me to work. The point is that most people consider it wrong to see another person's value as merely consisting in their usefulness to others in this kind of way. No researcher is likely to be devoid of ordinary human concerns such as compassion but the pressure of the research agenda may weaken such concerns and introduce a degree of ambiguity about exactly how the research participant is being perceived.

It could be argued that where mutuality is preserved, action research offers a collaborative venture from engagement to publication, and thus escapes from the means–ends dilemma of research. However, one might want to be circumspect about this claim, for even in the most cooperative of enterprises, for example, the cooperative inquiry group (Reason, 1988) difficulties may emerge. Academic researchers may need to produce a final report for publication whereas other group members may have a preference for simply remembering the experience. The work of producing final formulations may therefore suit some and not others in the group (Reason, 1988, p. 37). Related to this is the issue of "stakeholders" (those who can be considered to "have a stake" in the research process) referred to by Guba and Lincoln (1989). A democratic view requires that such research (termed "evaluation" in their paradigm) should consider the stakes that all the stakeholders have in the evaluation process and that fairness should be seen to operate. In hierarchical organisations, as Lathlean aptly describes, this is a very tricky if not impossible task to accomplish since the true collaborators are those who invited the researchers in. By definition, not everyone in the organisation has equal power to influence the invitation. Rapoport makes some observations concerning the management of this kind of difficulty in industry when he says:

> . . . information is sometimes sought and used in the context of industrial conflict. This issue is dealt with in a number of our projects nowadays by making an explicit agreement that though the financing of a project will lie with management, information provided will also be available to labour (Rapoport, 1970, p. 504).

Benefits and Harms

Johnson and Plant (p. 93) make the important observation that these need to be considered together because "what appeared to be a cost to one participant was of benefit to another". This of course means that the impact of the research on individuals is virtually impossible to predict in advance and thus presents an obvious difficulty in seeking consent. Such researchers often speak of the need to renegotiate consent at intervals; a process which may be compounded by the loyalties and attachments that gradually develop between researcher and participant. The language of "costs" is also interesting because if I judge that the costs were worth it, then I would not consider that I have been harmed, but if I say "it was far too costly" this would certainly convey regret at my involvement and some sense of resulting threat and/or damage. Johnson and Plant's study is the only one that describes instances, albeit only a few, where the research process could be said to have had an adverse effect on participants. The honesty and clarity with which this is expressed will hopefully enliven professional debate on this subject.

Lützén and Buckingham give powerful expression to the idea of possible harm resulting from the research process but in terms of omissions (rightful acts not done) rather than commissions (wrongful acts done). The distinction between these two becomes rather fragile in a context of a duty of care, as in a profession, for then rightful acts not done can sometimes be seen to be just as bad morally as wrongful acts committed. For example, if I deliberately neglect to feed my children and they starve to death (omission) this would not be regarded as in any sense morally preferable to smothering them to death (commission). We would, however, tend to think that my not giving money to a beggar in the street and his subsequent death from starvation (which I read about in the newspaper) while likely to provoke guilt in me and possible moral censure by others, will not provoke the same moral reaction as if I had killed the person. Not everyone is convinced by the usefulness of the "omission"/ "commission" distinction for moral analysis and someone could claim that what is morally determinative in the above example concerns the nature of the relationships we have with each other. Family relationships involving dependency and intimacy are simply not viewed morally in the same way as encounters between strangers.

Nevertheless, and regardless of which moral description one gives to these events, it is important both morally and professionally, to wonder which of these two scenarios best reflects the position of the nurse-researcher. Is such a person more like a stranger in the encounter with participants or more like someone in a defined relationship where there is a clearly understood duty of care? It may be argued that in certain contexts, unless research is overtly accompanied by a programme of change to which everyone involved has subscribed, it should not be carried out. Since, however, data have to be gathered before problems can be understood, even this view does not dispense with the moral disquiet of witnessing bad practice and not doing anything about it immediately.

In the context of action research described by Lathlean, the whole concept of what might be considered to be constructive, as opposed to destructive change underpins the justification of doing this work. It is inherently morally normative, containing within it some picture or series of pictures about what good change would amount to. Since not everyone's visions may be the same on this matter, preliminary discussion and agreement on an "ethical framework" is required for this sort of work (Rapoport, 1970, p. 499). However, as Lathlean (p. 35) observes "any early agreement as such was somewhat superficial and implicit rather than explicit". This would seem inevitable in a context where people cannot accurately foresee what is going to happen, so there may be limited imagination about the nature of any moral dilemmas which may subsequently present. This would mean that in reality people have to think on their feet and one would wonder if it is not the most powerful source of influence (whether researcher or manager or some combination) which dictates the vision of what a "good change" will be.

Whatever the difficulties and limitations, it may still be preferable to have tried to establish a "mutually acceptable ethical framework" in advance, and while action research is the only research process to have made this idea definitional, other research approaches might benefit from using it. It is possible that the painful dilemmas that Sylvia Buckingham experienced could have been managed with less personal cost to the researcher, if they had been anticipated and such thinking had been built into the original consent-seeking process. It must be no coincidence that Miller and Evans (1991, p. 380) and Kim Lützén arrive at the same conclusion, and Lützén states in her recommendations for the future:

> Careful preparation should include discussing with the people to be studied the possibility that certain fieldwork observations might be interpreted as bad practice. Discuss with the staff how to deal with this possibility (Lützén, p. 83).

For all the difficulties, it has to be said that many participants in the research described obviously gained a great deal from the research process and such gains ranged from the "spin off" of a protocol for skin care that Watson (p. 14) refers to, to the career advice provided by Rogers (p. 26) and the cathartic experiences felt to be beneficial by many of the people in Ersser's and Johnson and Plant's work. One interpretation of the gifts that Johnson and Plant (p. 95) received would be to see them as spontaneous responses from people who felt "given to" by the researchers. However, such gains cannot provide a justification for doing research since if we seriously thought this, we might be forced to conclude that, in the interests of patient care, all patients should not only have a named nurse but also a named researcher! As Kodish *et al.* observe, concerning randomised controlled trials:

> . . . if the argument is valid that patients have more hope and receive better care in RCT protocols, this should be taken not so much as a defense of RCT's but as an indictment of routine medical care (Kodish *et al.*, 1991, p. 182).

Nevertheless, neither should one dismiss the altruistic motives that many people may express in wishing to participate in research and the satisfaction that they may feel in contributing in this way. For those who are terminally ill, this motivation may be even more compelling with the involvement in research becoming a bequest to a future generation (Benoliel, 1980, p. 127).

Publication and Confidentiality

Benefits and harms are not just limited to the process of the research but are also consequences of publication. Buckingham (pp. 68) for instance expresses great concern about the possibly damaging consequences of conveying unexpected data which would have singled out a particular group of nurses as being deficient in their ability to assess children in pain. Things have to be seen in context and nurses with this particular qualification were having their training phased out and were expected to "convert" to registered nursing during the period that the research was conducted. Such practitioners might, therefore, already have had some reason to feel stigmatised and disadvantaged. The unexpected nature of this discovery also meant that consent had not been obtained to share this kind of material. As Rogers (p. 30) observes: "Any kind of research can expose a disparity between reality and some rule or ideal and so cause trouble" but she suggests this needs to be balanced beside the view that ". . . if respondents have given their time, the research team have worked on the data and the funding organisation have monitored the research throughout, the results should be published and not suppressed" (p. 29). In two projects data were checked with participants either partially (Rogers) or completely (Lathlean) prior to publication, and it is interesting that in the phase of initiating the research Watson (p. 6) made sure that all the companies involved in supplying equipment knew that the results would be published. Ersser (p. 53) took great trouble to explain to participants that "all data would remain anonymous and confidential" but "sought their permission to use a limited amount of anonymous printed data". He raises the question of whether or not the data provider should have the final say and be able to ask for confidential information to be destroyed (p. 53), as recommended by the National Institute for Nursing, 1993) and he addresses the issue of the need to inform participants of the outcomes of the study.

In ethnographic research, there is an obvious difficulty concerning the preservation of confidentiality. It is not difficult to offer apparent anonymity via the use of pseudonyms but, in small groups of people, individuals may be easily recognisable to others from their use of typical expressions or attitudes. This can cause considerable distress and is a potential problem, for example, in family research Larrossa *et al.*, 1981, p. 309). One also has to remember that the impact of the printed word is different from the verbal and people may be shocked by the sight of their own words staring at them from the paper (Sandelowski, 1993, p. 6). Lathlean tackled this difficulty directly but at the possible expense of producing a rather "bland" report (Lathlean, pp. 39–40). This may not have been too crucial for a style of research where the process of creating change is of at least as much value as reports of ultimate outcomes.

The sheer complexity of issues that may arise in deciding to agree data for publication with research participants is well documented by Sandelowski (1993). She observes, for example, that:

> Both members [research participants] and researchers are interested in accounts that represent experience fairly, but they may have very different views concerning what a fair account is (Sandelowski, 1993, p. 5).

For similar reasons, it would be important to discuss confidentiality at the time of gaining access because it may be that the research participants and the researcher have rather different pictures concerning what this in fact entails. For those who equate confidentiality with secrecy, the publication of any information beyond the statistical may be perceived as a breach but, for those who feel satisfied by anonymity, the publication of narrative excerpts may pose no problem. Some people may consider that the supervision the researcher receives constitutes a threat to confidentiality, others might be relieved to know that there is a supervisor. Questions clearly arise as to who is to be regarded as a member of the research team for the purposes of storing and sharing information and whether or not the participant knows this. Nurse-researchers who have worked as nurses in the National Health Service may have come to take for granted a particular picture of confidentiality which they unquestioningly continue to promote in the research context. The notion of "The NHS Family" which serves to underpin an NHS document on the subject of confidentiality (Department of Health, 1992) might be considered to be morally troubling by some people. It is far from obvious that one of the largest employers in Europe is appropriately to be seen as a "family", but one feature of a family structure is that more information is shared within the structure than is judged appropriate to divulge outside it. It might, therefore, serve as a convenient metaphor for making the sharing of information sound benign in a context where much of what is taken for granted should possibly be questioned (Kennedy, 1994).

Reassuring potential research participants about confidentiality raises the question of the power of the researcher to offer genuine guarantees. One wonders, for example, in the case of Lützén (p. 77) where she reassured people "that the data collected were not going to be used by the administration for the evaluation of staff performance" how she could be certain about this when the chief of staff was her research adviser.

Termination

It might be assumed that the termination of the research occurs at the point of publication, but with those studies that engage with people in a prolonged way, such that a relationship can be said to have formed, there is the issue of ending these relationships. It is a subject to which general nursing tends to give too little attention in clinical care, so it is unlikely that thinking on this matter will be widespread among the community of research nurses. Johnson and Plant (p. 97) make an important observation on this issue: "In some instances the problem of disengagement continued long after the project had been completed and to this day both of us still have contact with one or two participants." This continuation of contact might be welcomed by all parties but, on the other hand, it might become burdensome for researchers and involve unrealistic expectations from participants concerning what the researchers can continue to offer. Such relationships could conceivably even get in the way of people seeking more appropriate sources of help and support. Dingwall observes:

> Individuals may develop a degree of dependence on the research which advances data collection but which is not necessarily in their own best interests and may lead to abuse (Dingwall, 1980, p. 882).

In the sensitive work described, I see nothing that I would want to call "abuse" but if, as has already been suggested, "feeling understood" tends to promote attachment, the more sensitive and compassionate the researcher is, the more the issue of ending and parting will need to be addressed. In a therapeutic relationship, it is worked towards with space given to consider the feelings of loss that are generated. Accepting offers of hospitality probably needs to be understood from this sort of perspective. Does it feel entirely comfortable and would a refusal be merely churlish, or is it indicative of confusion in the minds of participants and part of an attempt to "make friends" with the researcher? There are clearly no rules to follow here, but judgement is required and preferably judgement that understands how the research process may invite dependency.

In conclusion, I would simply like to endorse the experience of Johnson and Plant in their search for a form of supervision which would enable the complexities of the interactions they were involved in to be understood and which could facilitate their ability to make good judgements or at least better ones. For those kinds of research which use a reflexive approach, it could also be said to be indispensable to the method (Laslett and Rapoport, 1975, pp. 970–971). Recognising the essential need for this kind of support would require that it be planned and budgeted for when designing the research.

References

Benoliel, J.Q. (1980) Research with dying patients. In Davis, A.J. and Krueger, J.C. (eds) *Patients, Nurses Ethics*, Chapter 11. New York: American Journal of Nursing Co.

Borbasi, S. (1994) To be or not to be? Nurse? Researcher? Or both? *Nursing Inquiry*, **1**, 57.

Department of Health (1992) *Confidentiality, Use and Disclosure of N.H.S. Information: Health Service Guidelines*. London: Department of Health.

Dingwall, R. (1980) Ethics and ethnography. *Sociological Review*, **28**(4), 871–891.

Guba, E.C. and Lincoln, Y.S. (1989) *Fourth generation evaluation*. Newbury Park, California: Sage Publications.

Heron, J. (1988) Validity in co-operative inquiry. In Reason, P. (ed.) *Human Inquiry in Action*, Chapter 2. London: Sage Publications.

Kennedy, I. (1994) Guest editorial: between ourselves. *Journal of Medical Ethics*, **20**, 69–70, 100.

Kodish, E., Lantos, J.D. and Siegler, M. (1991) Opinion: the ethics of randomisation. *CA-A Cancer Journal for Clinicians*, **41**(3), 180–186.

Larossa, R., Bennett, L. and Gelles, R. (1981) Ethical dilemmas in qualitative family research. *Journal of Marriage and the Family*, **43**(2), 303–313.

Laslett, B. and Rapoport, R. (1975) Collaborative interviewing and interactive research. *Journal of Marriage and the Family*, **37** (Nov), 968–977.

May, K.A. (1979) The nurse as researcher: impediment to informed consent? *Nursing Outlook*, **27**(1), 36–39.

Miller, J. and Evans, T. (1991) Some reflections on ethical dilemmas in nursing home research. *Western Journal of Nursing Research*, **13**(3), 375–380.

Munhall, P.L. (1988) Ethical considerations in qualitative research. *Western Journal of Nursing Research*, **10**(2), 150–162.

National Institute of Nursing (1993) *Code of Conduct for Researchers*. National Institute for Nursing, Radcliffe Infirmary, Oxford, UK.

Rapoport, R.N. (1970) Three dilemmas in action research. *Human Relations*, **23**(6), 499–513.

Reason, P. (ed.) (1988) *Human Inquiry in Action*. London: Sage Publications.

Robertson, J.A. (1991) Second thoughts on living wills. *Hastings Center Report*, **21**(6), 6–9.

Royal College of Nursing (1993) *Ethics related to research in nursing*. Harrow: Scutari Press.

Sandelowski, M. (1993) Rigor or rigor mortis: the problem of rigor in qualitative research revisited. *Advances in Nursing Science*, **16**(2), 1–8.

Smith, L. (1992) Ethical issues in interviewing. *Journal of Advanced Nursing*, **17**, 98–103.

9

Legal Issues

Bridgit Dimond

The conduct of research is not without legal implications and before the researcher commences any work, he or she should be mindful of the legal dimensions. The main topics which will be considered in this chapter are as follows, though it is accepted that this list is not exhaustive:

(1) laws and international covenants;
(2) prohibited areas;
(3) consent;
(4) confidentiality;
(5) negligence;
(6) control over publication.

1. Laws and International Covenants

What is the law and how is it enforced?

The law in the UK is created in two main ways: either through statutory provision or by the judges in the courts making decisions in cases which can then be used as precedents in subsequent cases. Statutory provision consists of primary legislation, e.g. Acts of Parliament, including legislation from the European Community, and secondary legislation, which includes statutory instruments and directions which are enacted by those authorised in the primary legislation.

European Union law

Following the UK's signing of the Treaty of Rome and the UK joining the European Union (EU), the UK is bound by the laws issued by the Council of Ministers and the European Commission and by the rulings by the European Court of Justice in Luxembourg. There is no appeal against its decisions. Increasingly, where there is a doubt about the interpretation of European Law, the English Court will refer a series of questions to the European Court of Justice on an issue before it, prior to making a decision on the merits of the case.

Regulations issued by the EU are mandatory. They have automatic force throughout the EU. Directives are binding as to the aim to be achieved but the actual choice of methods of compliance are left to individual states. Legislation by each state is therefore necessary. Decisions are rulings in individual cases which are binding upon individuals or organisations.

The EU has been principally concerned with the removal of barriers to trade and freedom of movement of goods and persons within the EU. However, the acceptance of the Social Charter by 11 of the 12 member states in 1991 (The UK's refusal to accept the Social Charter was recognised by the other member states) will lead to an increasing concern with the individual conditions and rights of employees.

European Commission Directive 91/507/EEC

The directive requires member states to conform to good clinical practice in carrying out trials on medicinal products before seeking authorisation for marketing. It also requires that the clinical trial shall conform to the ethical principles set out in the current Declaration of Helsinki (see Appendix). The freely informed consent of each trial subject must be obtained and documented.

This directive became binding in this country on 1 January 1992 and explicitly gives legal force to the declaration of Helsinki. Regulation has not yet been passed for its implementation within this country.

Charter of Human Rights and the United Nations

This Charter, established in 1945, contains a declaration relating to belief in "the fundamental human rights, in the dignity and worth of the human person, in the dignity of men and women and of nations large and small" and in the promotion of the observation of these beliefs. It also provided for the establishment of a Commission on Human Rights.

Universal Declaration of Human Rights

The Commission on Human Rights of the United Nations had as its first task the preparation of an International Bill of Rights. This was proclaimed by the General Assembly of the United Nations in 1948 as a Universal Declaration of Human Rights and was followed in 1966 by three additional international treaties covering:

(1) International Covenant on Economic, Social and Cultural Rights;
(2) International Covenant on Civil and Political Rights;
(3) the Optional Protocol creating right of communication and petition.

The Covenant provided for the establishment of an international organisation called the Human Rights Committee which considers applications relating to infringements of rights and then forwards its views to the state concerned and to the individual.

The European Convention for the Protection of Human Rights and Fundamental Freedoms

This was signed first in 1950 and took as its starting point the Universal Declaration of Human Rights. The Convention is accepted in 26 member countries of the Council of Europe (Beddard, 1993). It is estimated that more than 450 million persons in Europe may bring before the European Commission of Human Rights allegations that their rights have been violated. Up to the end of 1991, 19 000 cases had been through the Commission. It must be distinguished from the Court of Justice of the EU which only covers those member states which have specifically agreed and been allowed to join. The European Commission meets in Strasbourg. It is accepted that its decision and the declaration itself has had immense influence upon the European Court of Justice of the EU in Luxembourg.

The UK and the European Convention of Human Rights

It should be noted, however, that whilst the UK is a signatory to the Convention, its principles are not automatically legally binding in this country. Nor is there in the UK a Bill of Rights which sets out, like the Bill of Rights of the USA, a declaration of the fundamental rights of each individual in the state which are enforceable in every court. Instead, the person who alleges a breach of a fundamental right in the UK must point to actual legislation, primary or secondary (either from the UK or from the EU) or to the decision in a comparable case which is relevant and would be binding in his particular circumstances, in order to enforce the right. This is why in the following discussion concerning the law in the UK, statutes and cases will be quoted to show which specific laws are relevant to the researcher and which are directly enforceable in this country. The declaration of rights by the United Nations and by the European Convention are not directly enforceable in the UK. However, the European Directive cited above is directly enforceable, even though the implementing regulations have not been passed.

Relationship between the law and ethics

Many professional bodies and international organisations have established Codes of Practice and protocols on the ethical issues arising in research. In the UK, the Royal College of Nursing Research Advisory Group (RCN, 1993) has prepared and revised a paper on the ethics related to research in nursing. This establishes a helpful framework for nurse practitioners, whether they are actually conducting research themselves or caring for patients who are asked to be involved in research. However, it should be recognised that these principles of ethics are not necessarily a statement of what the law would recognise as enforceable. For example, on confidentiality the RCN state as a principle that "any promises of anonymity or confidentiality given to the participants by the researcher must be respected . . .". However, there may be laws which override this duty of confidentiality (see below). This gap between principles of ethics and the law of each country is also true of some international codes (see Declaration of Helsinki principles 9 and 10 in the Appendix).

The rights enshrined in these principles are not directly enforceable in a court of law in the UK, but for the most part they are paralleled by laws which are recognised as enforceable.

2. Prohibited Areas

There will be some areas of research practice which would be defined as illegal. In the UK, for example, it would be illegal under the Human Fertilisation and Embryology Act 1990 to conduct research on an embryo after the development of the primitive streak (i.e. 14 days). It is also illegal to place in a woman a live embryo other than a human embryo or live gametes other than human gametes. In addition the House of Lords has made it clear that an individual cannot give a consent which would be accepted as a valid defence to an act which constituted an offence against the person such as sadomasochistic acts (R. v. Brown and others, 1993). Therefore the fact that subjects purported to give consent would not make legal research which would otherwise be illegal.

3. Consent

Research on subjects who have not consented arouses great consternation and is the heart of the dilemma of the conflict between paternalism (acting in the best interests of the patient without necessarily obtaining the patient's consent) and autonomy (allowing the patient the choice even though he or she chooses something which is not in his or her best interests). In the past there have been examples of over-zealous researchers who stepped beyond what was acceptable. The name Willowbrook (Beauchamp and Childress, 1989, p. 431), for example, is infamous: parents of severely mentally handicapped children who were desperate to find residential care for their children were given priority in the allocation of places if they agreed to their child taking part in a research project which involved the child being injected with a hepatitis virus.

In 1986 the Bulletin of Medical Ethics drew attention to an MRC research study which was undertaken to compare early or deferred orchiectomy (i.e. castration) in two categories of men with newly diagnosed prostatic cancer (Editorial, 1986). The editor suggested that the trial was of doubtful scientific value and was unethical in its conduct. Consent was not obtained from all patients, nor was full information about the trial given.

More recently the same journal highlighted the case of Mrs Evelyn Thomas (*Bulletin of Medical Ethics*, 1988a, b, 1992a) who alleged that she had been used in two trials for breast cancer without her knowledge or consent. One trial was of counselling for mastectomy patients and the other was of tamoxifen and cyclophosphamide as adjuvant chemotherapy in early breast cancer. Mrs Thomas eventually complained to the Health Service Commissioner about the delay in the handling of her complaint and about the dissemination of her personal medical data through various computer systems. In spite of her death, the Ombudsman continued the investigation and concluded that "patients are entitled to expect that confidential information about them is carefully safeguarded and that their identity is protected" and sought assurances from the health authority to that effect. In evidence to the Select Committee of the House of Commons the chairman of the Research Ethics Committee explained that subsequently they obtained full informed consent but at a different time, not immediately after the operation on the breast.

It is essential that before research commences, subjects give a full informed consent to the research being carried out. The areas of consent to research which will be covered in this paper are:

(a) mentally competent adults;
(b) (i)   children of 16 and 17 years;
    (ii) children under 16 years;
(c) mentally disordered minors;

(d) mentally disordered adults;
(e) withdrawal of consent;
(f) form in which consent should be given.

The nature of the consent which must be obtained depends to a certain extent on whether the research is regarded as therapeutic or non-therapeutic.

Definition of therapeutic and non-therapeutic research

These terms are frequently used in the context of research and are taken to imply that in therapeutic research the data subject stands to receive direct benefit from the research which is undertaken as part of his or her treatment. In one sense all treatment is potentially in the nature of research, since all professionals should stand to learn lessons from the effect of treatment on any individual patient, even though the treatment is well tried and much used. In contrast, non-therapeutic research is conducted without any direct or indirect benefit to the data subject.

In the case of Re F (F v. West Berkshire HA, 1989) the House of Lords refused to draw a distinction between a sterilisation for therapeutic purposes (e.g. cancer etc.) and one for non-therapeutic purposes (e.g. to prevent pregnancy on social grounds) and in the context of the issue before them (whether a mentally handicapped woman incapable of giving consent should be sterilised) this was probably reasonable. However, in the context of research the distinction is important and significant to the question as to whether paternalism can ever have a part to play in consent to research. For example, a patient might be offered a place on a trial for a new drug which has a good chance of being better that those currently being prescribed. Where the research can be considered to be of direct benefit to the patient, it may be appropriate to withhold certain information from the patient as is considered possible in exceptional circumstances. See the case of Sidaway below (Sidaway v. Board of Governors of Royal Bethlem and Maudsley Hospital, 1985).

(a) Mentally competent adults

A mentally competent adult can give or refuse consent to treatment. Otherwise any touching of him or her is termed a "trespass to his/her person". A trespass is actionable without the person touched proving that any harm has occurred. The mere touching is a civil wrong, and is subject to compensation in the civil courts. Before consent to treatment is given, the law requires that the person is given sufficient information of significant risks of substantial harm to make a decision. However, the law does not require that all information is given to patients. The professional is entitled to exercise what is known as therapeutic privilege and withhold information which is likely to cause harm to the patient. The test applied to determine the standard of care in such circumstances is known as the "Bolam Test" (Bolam v. Friern Hospital Management Committee, 1957). This states that: "The test as to whether there has been negligence or not is . . . the standard of the ordinary skilled man exercising or professing to have that special care." The right at common law (i.e. judge-made law) for the professional to withhold information is mirrored by the statutory restrictions on access to health records whether contained in computer form or manually. In the former case, access is governed by the Data Protection Act 1984 and the regulations issued under that Act; in the latter case, access for manually held health records is governed by the Access to Health Records Act 1990. Both the 1984 Act and the 1990 Act have the same rights of exclusion of access.

That is the situation in respect to consent to treatment. Where consent to research participation is at issue, then it is submitted that the nature of the consent required depends upon whether the research is of any therapeutic benefit to the patient. It is suggested that where the research has therapeutic purposes, then similar provisions would apply as for consent to treatment and in exceptional circumstances it might be that the researcher would be entitled to withhold certain information from the patient, since the research has a therapeutic aim. Much, however, depends on the existence of alternative treatments and the reason for withholding information and the physical and mental condition of the patient.

In contrast, where the research has no therapeutic benefit to the patient, either directly or indirectly, then the researcher would have a duty to give the research subject all the relevant information which could influence the decision to consent to participation in the research programme. Forms for consent to research would be vetted by the local research ethics committee together with any written information about the research project which would be given to the subject before consent is requested.

In the Sidaway case, cited above, the House of Lords declared that the English law did not recognise a doctrine of informed consent if what was meant by that was that all information had to be given to the patient before consent was obtained. However, it could be said that in situations of non-therapeutic research, there may be an informed consent situation, since the subject is entitled to receive all relevant information before giving consent to participation.

Further issues arise in the giving of information about the research before consent is obtained where, at the beginning of the project, the researchers cannot be sure what are the potential risks and benefits of the research. Furthermore, the researchers may be unable to predict the effects which the research will actually have upon the patients themselves. It is difficult to obtain an informed consent in such circumstances.

Use of volunteers

To be valid, consent must be freely given without force or coercion. Researchers often rely heavily upon attracting volunteers to participate. However, whilst no full payment is offered the subject, there might be payment of generous travelling or subsistence expenses. Does this destroy the voluntary nature of the offer to assist and make the person a paid helper? If so is this change of relationship of any significance in law? Could the offer of reward in some way affect the validity of the consent?

It is possible that where inducements to take part in the research are substantial, there comes into being a contractual relationship between researcher and the subject. This would not necessarily invalidate the consent given by the subject but it might change the legal relationship of the researcher and subject, who might be seen as a paid employee.

(b) Children

(i) Children of 16 and 17 years

The Family Law Reform Act 1969 gives the 16- and 17-year-old the right to give consent to medical and dental treatment. The word treatment includes anaesthetic and diagnostic procedures. It does not give explicitly a statutory right for the minor of 16 and 17 to consent to participation in research. However, on the basis of the House of Lords decision in the Gillick case (Gillick v. West Norfolk and Wisbech AHA and the DHSS, 1985) and in keeping with the philosophy underlining the Children Act 1989 of maximum participation of children in decisions where they have the intelligence and maturity to make a valid decision, a researcher would probably be able to undertake research on the basis of the consent of a minor of 16 or 17 if he or she had the maturity and understanding to make a competent decision.

Section 8(3) of the Family Law Reform Act 1969 enables any other consent to treatment, which would have been valid before the passing of the Act to continue to be relied upon. Thus the parent's consent for treatment of a 16- or 17-year-old would be valid. However, since the Act is restricted to treatment, it would seem unwise to rely upon this provision in relation to non-therapeutic research on a 16- or 17-year-old. A better view would be that unless the 16- or 17-year-old is able to give consent on his/her own behalf to participation in non-therapeutic research, the research should not involve that person. In the case of therapeutic research, where the 16- or 17-year-old is unable or refuses to give consent, but the parents are prepared to give consent, it is a question of the benefits to be derived from the treatment and whether the refusal of the minor should be overridden. It would seem necessary for the court to become involved as happened in the case of Re W (1992) also known as Re J.

(ii) Children under 16 years

The Medical Research Council issued guidance on the ethical conduct of research on children in 1991 (*Bulletin of Medical Ethics*, 1992b). It suggested the following safeguards:

(1) Children should only take part in research if the relevant knowledge could not be obtained from adults.
(2) All projects must be approved by the appropriate LREC.
(3) They should either have given consent, or consent must have been given on their behalf by a parent or guardian.

Therapeutic research can be carried out only if in the parents' opinion the benefits likely to accrue to the child outweigh the possible risks of harm and participation is therefore in his or her best interests.

Non-therapeutic research should only be carried out if there is negligible risk to the child and it is therefore not against his or her interests.

When a child has sufficient understanding to consent, his or her consent should be sought. It would still be advisable to seek parental consent as well. The Department of Health (1991) in its guidelines for LRECs gives similar advice. Following the Gillick case more weight has been given to the ability of the under 16-year-old to give a valid consent. This has been reinforced by the Children Act 1989, which gives to the child who is of sufficient under-standing to make an informed decision the right to refuse to submit to a medical or psychiatric examination or other assessment (S.43(8) and S.44(7)) and to treatment (Schedule 3 paras 4(4a) and 5 (5a)).

The research guidelines for LRECs (Department of Health, 1991) recom-mend that research proposals should only involve children where it is abso-lutely essential to do so and the information required cannot be obtained using adult subjects. Different principles apply according to the age and mental capacity of the child.

Non-therapeutic research

If the child has the mental competence to understand the risks and purpose of the research, then it is possible that he/she could give a valid consent to participation in it. Where the risks are significant, it is unwise to rely upon the child's consent. Nor, however, in such circumstances could there be justifica-tion in the parents giving consent to submit the child to the possible risk of harm. A parent can only give consent to what is in the child's best interests and can it ever be said that non-therapeutic research which will have no direct or indirect benefit to the child but carries a risk, could be in the child's best interests? The alternative argument is that the child might benefit from an altruistic act by taking pleasure in contributing to the information obtained which will help others. This might be so, but it would be preferable for the child to consent in his/her own right, rather than for the parents to do so on his/her behalf.

The LREC guidelines state that those acting for the child can only legally give their consent provided that the intervention is for the benefit of the child: "If they are responsible for allowing the child to be subjected to any risk (other than one so insignificant as to be negligible) which is not for the benefit of that child, it could be said they were acting illegally." Also "It should be noted that the giving of consent by a parent or guardian cannot overrule the refusal of consent by a child who is competent to make that decision." This was written before the decision in Re W (a minor) where the refusal of a 16-year-old suffering from anorexia nervosa to have treatment was overruled by the court. However, where the minor's views in refusing to give consent to participation in a research project are overruled it would have to be shown that the therapeutic benefits of the research justified the intervention in the minor's best interests.

(c) Mentally disordered minors

Exactly the same rules would apply for the protection of these patients as apply in the case of minors under 16 years. If there is the possibility that they have the capacity to give consent to participation in research, then their consent could be given. It is unlikely, however, that the parents could give consent on their behalf unless there were clear therapeutic benefits to the person from the research.

(d) Mentally disordered adults

The Law Commission (1991, 1993) has recommended legislation which would lead to provision being made for decisions on a variety of topics to be taken on behalf of the mentally incapacitated adult. However, participation in a research project where there are risks to the subject and minimal or no benefits is unlikely to be in the best interests of the person and, therefore, it is unlikely that any individual would have the authority to give consent on behalf of the mentally incapacitated adult. Reference to a judicial forum would be required.

Roger Watson (Chapter 1) describes the problem in relation to consent in his testing of incontinence products. He discusses the possibility of obtaining consent by proxy. Unfortunately, however, at present there is no power in law for a proxy to give consent to treatment or care on behalf of the mentally handicapped adult. The professional must act in the best interests of the patient, following the Bolam Test described previously.

The piloting of new drugs on mentally disordered persons has sometimes been carried out on the basis of a consent given by a local research ethics committee where patients are unable to give consent in their own right. This situation would be covered by the Law Commission proposals and, in the meantime, precautions should be taken to ensure that any such treatment is clearly in the best interests of each individual patient. In the case of Re F (F v. West Berkshire HA, 1989) the House of Lords stated that if a professional acted in the best interests of a person unable to give consent and followed the accepted approved standard of care, then he/she would not be acting unlawfully. However, it is unlikely that this dictum would cover the lack of any consent to research unless the research was therapeutically in the interests of the patient. Reference should be made to the guidelines issued by the Royal College of Psychiatrists.

It must not be assumed that because a person is mentally disordered, it automatically follows that he/she lacks the capacity to give a valid consent or refusal to participation in a research project. Thus, in a recent case, a patient in Broadmoor Special Hospital, who was suffering from gangrene, was able to obtain an injunction to prevent the hospital arranging for the amputation of his leg without his written consent. In spite of his paranoid schizophrenia, he was able to make a competent decision on refusing life-saving treatment (Re C, 1994).

As a matter of good practice it is recommended that where the consent of a person who is mentally disordered arises, a person other than the researcher should confirm the capacity of the patient to give a valid consent.

(e) Withdrawal of consent

It is essential that the patient should be notified at the time of giving consent to participation in a research project from which he/she stands to benefit therapeutically, that the person can withdraw at any time without any victimisation or any threat to his/her continued alternative treatment for that condition. This is emphasised in the RCN guidelines (1993): "The rights of refusal and withdrawal must be totally respected by researchers."

There is a danger that persons who depend upon the researchers for their continued health care may be under pressure to continue participation in the research. If there is any danger as a result of sudden cessation of treatment the patient should be warned of that possibility. There is also a danger that staff will be pressurised into testing out products or carrying out other research on their patients. Judith Lathlean (Chapter 3) queries that: "since all newly appointed ward sisters . . . were automatically included in the programme, was there truly an element of choice?" (p. 38).

(f) Form of consent

Before giving its views on a research project, the LREC would normally expect to see the written form on which the consent is to be given. There is in fact no legal requirement for consent to be given in writing, but it is preferable if the research subject has that opportunity.

Ersser (Chapter 4), in discussing the autonomy of participants, states that: "The consent sought was of a verbal nature. At the time I felt the formality surrounding the use of a written consent form would risk generating suspicion. However, today I feel that gaining written consent would be desirable practice. A verbal explanation of the purpose of the research was also provided at the first meeting" (p. 47). There is a twofold danger here. The first is that the data subject does not really put his or her mind to the fact that he or she is giving consent to the research if it is obtained by word of mouth and the information about the research is also given by word of mouth. Can it really be said that there is real consent by the subject?

The second danger is that if there is eventually a conflict between the researcher and the subject over whether consent was actually given, it is one person's word against another, and written consent is preferable as evidence. In addition, if information about the project is given both by word of mouth and in writing, then it can be clearly established that the information was in fact given.

4. Confidentiality

Data subjects are entitled to the same duty of care in relation to confidentiality that they can expect from those health professionals who care for them. Unless, therefore, they give consent to the disclosure of personal information which is obtained by the researcher as a result of the research, the information must be kept confidential or used in a way which does not disclose the identity of the data subject. There are, however, exceptions to this principle and they are probably similar to those exceptions which apply in the therapeutic context.

Examples of conflicts over confidentiality are as follows.

(1) Through blood tests, a researcher discovers information of great potential interest to third parties, e.g. paternity issues, HIV status, genetic predisposition to disease, etc.
(2) A patient discovers that research has taken place, and the findings show that he or she has been treated negligently; the patient wishes to have access to these research findings to establish his or her claim for compensation.
(3) A researcher discovers a study that has already been carried out in his or her own field; the researcher wishes to prevent his/her subjects from suffering from the same side-effects which took place in that study and therefore asks the researchers to pass on this information to him/her.
(4) A researcher wishes to identify case studies of patients suffering from the

same condition and match them up in terms of personal attributes, which would have the effect of identifying the research subjects.

(5) A researcher discovers crime (fraud or other offences) during research.

Possible exceptions to the principle of confidentiality are:

(1) public interest, e.g. suspected child abuse;
(2) court order – the only information which cannot be ordered to be produced by the court is that covered by the public interest against disclosure and that covered by legal professional privilege;
(3) transfer of information between researchers;
(4) medical education;
(5) statutory requirements;
(6) disclosure with the consent of the patient.

All the above situations could be lawfully recognised as exceptions to the duty of confidentiality in the treatment context, and it is likely that there would be no distinction drawn between information obtained from the treatment situation and that obtained from the research situation.

The Department of Health (1994) has published a paper on "Confidentiality" which states that records based purely on research do not require the patient's consent, provided that:

(1) The LREC has advised that identifiable information may be used for the particular project and is satisfied with the arrangement proposed to safeguard patient confidentiality.
(2) The NHS body has decided that disclosure for the research can be justified in the public interest. However, no legal authority is claimed for this statement and it may be framed too widely with a much wider definition of public interest than the registration bodies, such as the UKCC, have used.

Confidentiality means the respect of information personal to the patient or data subject. As far as the law is concerned, there is no absolute right of access to health information held about a person. Whether the records are held on computer or in manual form, the information can be withheld if serious harm would be caused to the physical or mental health of the applicant. Staff also need to ensure that confidential information received is protected. Thus Jill Rogers (Chapter 2) points out the nurse's concern that "their comments about access to distance learning and continuing education opportunities could be disclosed to their managers". Clearly, however, it may be difficult to draft the research findings' report without identifying specific informants.

5. Negligence

Areas to be considered include:

(a) standard of care in research and the duty to inform;
(b) vicarious liability and the researcher;
(c) defences –
   (i)   contributory negligence,
   (ii)   *volenti non fit injuria,*
   (iii) exclusion of liability;
(d) compensation –
   (i)   *ex gratia* compensation,
   (ii)   indemnity,
   (iii) insurance cover and the researcher.

(a) Standard of care in research and the duty to inform

The test for the standard of care expected in the treatment and care of patients is known as the Bolam Test (described previously). It rests upon a concept of what the reasonable professional would have done in those circumstances following the accepted approved practice. However, it is difficult to apply this test in the area of research, when events may take place which are not reasonably foreseeable. In spite of this, in the event of an action being brought for compensation against a researcher or his/her employers for harm which has been caused during the research, in the absence of any statutory provision for no fault or strict liability to be available for volunteers, there is probably no other way of establishing that the researcher was negligent than in applying the Bolam Test.

The injured subject would therefore have to show that the researcher owed him/her a duty of care (which would probably be accepted), that the researcher failed to exercise the appropriate standard of care in relation to his/her safety and that, as a foreseeable consequence, harm has been caused to the subject.

Failure to warn the subject of foreseeable risks of harm would also be actionable in negligence, but to obtain compensation the plaintiff (i.e. the person bringing the action) would have to show not only the breach of care but also that the failure to warn led the subject to participate and suffer those risks of which he should have been warned.

Negligence and the observer/researcher

Buckingham (Chapter 5) raises an extremely important legal issue concerning the duty of the observer/researcher when he or she witnesses unacceptable practice: "I had a greater knowledge of the child and his previous medical history than the nurse caring for him. I wanted to challenge her on the way that she had allowed the mother to make decisions regarding the child's pain" (p. 65) and "Should I intervene or should I allow the nurse to decide?" (p. 66) are examples of the conflict which arose.

To my knowledge there is no decided case directly on the point of whether the researcher has a duty to intervene. One could take the view that he or she is not on the ward in his or her capacity as a professional practitioner and does not have a duty of care towards the patients in a professional capacity and the law does not require him/her to volunteer his/her services. Therefore, the researcher could stand by and watch children suffering unnecessary discomfort and pain with no legal duty to intervene.

The alternative view is that the researcher is a professional practitioner and has a duty defined by the UKCC in its Code of Professional Conduct. Even though this is not legally enforceable in the courts, failure to observe the Code could lead to the practitioner facing professional conduct proceedings for misconduct (defined as "conduct unworthy of a nurse, midwife and health visitor"). There would be circumstances in which the needs of the research could not take priority over the care of the patient. For example, in a situation where the observer saw an unattended child about to fall through an open window, there would probably be both a professional and a legal duty for the researcher to prevent the child's death.

The conflicts which can arise and which are so clearly described by Sylvia Buckingham need to be further debated from a legal and professional standpoint. The RCN (1993, p. 8) advice is directly in point: "Any nurse researcher must decide at what point ethical requirements necessitate an intervention in order to maintain the safety of the patients/clients, whatever the consequences for the research . . . this could include abandoning data collection in that area . . .". The ethical situation may be clear but there are no decided cases on the point. Judith Lathlean also describes very clearly the tensions for the researchers in knowing when to intervene and use their power.

Legal significance of research and the duty of care for the future

Professional practice should be research based. It is not, however, always easy to determine the stage at which the standards of care are changed to incorporate the research findings. To what extent does the professional have a duty to take note of the research findings of others? There will always be a delay before the results of research projects are incorporated in revised standards of care. The courts do not expect practice to change immediately a paper is published advising such a change.

In one case a patient developed brachial palsy during a blood transfusion. An article had appeared in the *Lancet* six months previously describing this hazard (Crawford v. Charing Cross Hospital, 1953). The patient lost the case on the grounds that provided the professional staff were following the accepted approved practice at that time (now known as the Bolam Test), then it could not be said that they were negligent in failing to apply or be aware of recent knowledge. Obviously the extent to which research findings must be followed will depend upon their status: an announcement from the Committee for the Safety of Medicines would have immediate effect upon standards of practice.

(b) Vicarious liability

Sometimes the researcher is undertaking research in the course of his/her employment. In such cases the employer would be vicariously liable for any harm which occurred to the subject as a result of the negligence of the researcher. This does not apply where the researcher is undertaking research as a private personal project, which is not done on behalf of his/her employer.

The researcher should clarify, before the work commences, the involvement or interest of his employer. This is particularly so where he/she is likely to be involved in the research during working hours or where he/she is likely to be using information from the workplace as part of the research. The employer would have the right to refuse permission and therefore, his/her authority to proceed should be sought. This is considered below in relation to the control of the research outcomes.

(c) Defences to an action for negligence

(i) Contributory negligence

A defence to an action for negligence is that the plaintiff or person claiming compensation was him/herself at fault and so he/she was partly to blame for his/her pain and suffering or other loss. This defence is known as contributory negligence. The defendant would have to establish that the plaintiff was in breach of the duty which he owes to him/herself. An example would be where research subjects are advised at the beginning to pass on any information which would be relevant to the research, e.g. any special aspects of their present health and any medications which they were taking, or to inform the researcher immediately of any side-effects of the research. If the subject deliberately concealed this information from the researcher and, as a result of this concealment, the research caused him/her harm then there would be a reduction of any compensation payable because of this contributory negligence. Clearly, when considering whether the subject has been contributorily negligent, account would be taken of the capacity of the subject to understand the instructions and to comply with them. In such circumstances, the written evidence of what information was given to the subject about disclosure would be vital. In some research projects it would be incumbent upon the researcher to obtain, with the consent of the subject, clinical information from the subject's medical practitioner before the research could commence.

(ii) Volenti non fit injuria

Another defence is the possibility of claiming that the subject agreed to take part in the research and therefore waived any right to claim compensation when something went wrong. If this defence is to succeed, it would have to be established that the subject clearly agreed to all the risks and that these were explained to him and that he gave a clear consent to take them. If the researcher has been negligent and risks occur which have not been accepted by the subject the researcher would be liable.

(iii) Exclusion of liability

The researcher cannot attempt to exclude his liability for negligence by requiring the subject to sign a paper to that effect. This is because of the provisions of the Unfair Contract Terms Act 1977 which prevents anyone exempting themselves from liability for their negligence where this causes personal injury or death. Liability for loss or damage of property can be excluded if the exclusion can be shown to be reasonable.

(d) Forms of compensation payment

(i) Ex gratia *payments*

The Pearson Report (1978) recommended that *ex gratia* payments should be made to those injured in research activities, but this recommendation has never been enacted in law. Nevertheless, many pharmaceutical companies recognise a duty to pay out compensation to those injured during research, and this is payable without the victim having to establish fault. This is made clear to participants when they give consent to take part.

(ii) Indemnity

Sometimes in large research studies financed by an institution or company, the organisation responsible for initiating the research agrees that in the event of any harm occurring, even without negligence, then an indemnity will be paid to the researcher for any loss or harm which is suffered by the subject. Sometimes, this payment might be offered direct to the research subject. If participation is undertaken in a research project and it is agreed that the payment of an indemnity would be made then this would be a binding contract enforceable against the person offering the indemnity, since the subject has given the consideration of his/her involvement in the research as his/her part of the bargain.

(iii) Insurance cover

Whether or not the researcher is advised to obtain insurance cover depends upon the potential risks of the research and who, if anyone, is financing it. If, for example, the researcher might face the threat of legal action because of the results being invalid, therefore causing financial loss to others, this might not be a loss which the funding body is prepared to accept and it would hold the researcher responsible since it was the inadequacies of the research which caused the errors.

Insurance might also be necessary where personal accidents to the researchers might occur.

6. Publication

Controls over publication

The various organisations which might attempt to control the publishing of the research are:

(a) employers who have/have not funded research;
(b) outside funding body;
(c) other interested parties;
(d) Higher Education institution;
(e) clinical location where the research took place.

It is essential that the researcher should, even before the research commences, identify who is to have the legal property in the research and the control over its publication. If this is agreed, then censorship from those who feel uncomfortable at the research findings may be prevented. It does not necessarily follow that the funding body will automatically have the right to censor the research and control publication. It depends upon the nature of the agreement when the funding was arranged. Jill Rogers (Chapter 2) brings out very clearly the issues relating to the presentation of results and the control over publication. It is essential that these issues are clarified before the research begins.

It may be significant that the research is done outside of working hours if the employer is claiming the controls over the research or rights to obtain the benefits.

Potential problems arising from publication

What if research findings result in the condemnation of other therapies etc., causing financial loss, and then the research is itself criticised and dis-counted? An example of such a situation is the criticism of the Bristol Cancer Help Centre, as a result of research which did not take into account the fact that the patients going to that centre were far more ill than patients going to other centres. The facts were that research published in the *Lancet* in 1990 claimed that women with breast cancer who supplemented their treatment with alternative therapy were twice as likely to die as those who received conventional treatment alone. There was a direct reference to the Bristol Cancer Help Centre which provided such treatment. However, two months after this research was published the researchers admitted that they did not take into account the differences in the severity of the cancer of the two groups, since those at the Bristol Centre had had more advanced disease. As a result of this adverse research, patients stopped attending the Centre, which suffered considerable financial loss. It is unknown at the present time whether legal action is being taken in respect of the faulty research, but in theory there could be a duty of care owed by researchers to those who suffer harm as a reasonably foreseeable consequence of a breach of the duty of care.

In another criticism of a research project (*The Times*, 1993) it was reported that the Institute for Cancer Research was taking legal action over the right to sue for libel claiming scientific fraud. A report by an expert advisory group on the research capabilities of the Royal Marsden Hospital was described by the cancer experts as incompetent and so irresponsible as possibly to consti-tute professional misconduct.

The lesson for researchers, whatever the outcome in the above examples, is that the appropriate standards of care must be followed at every stage of the research project in order to ensure that no successful action for negligence or negligent mis-statement can be brought.

Conclusions

This discussion does not necessarily cover all the potential legal issues which arise from research. However, it was the intention to point out to the re-searcher some of the potential hazards which should be borne in mind when research is contemplated. It should not, however, discourage the practitioner from carrying out research since all practice should be research based. It hopefully provides guidance for the protection of both the research subject and the researcher. Ultimately, in any conflict between the two the interests of the subject must prevail.

Concern for the interests of the subject must always prevail over the interests of science, society and the researcher (see Declaration of Helsinki: Principle 5 in the Appendix).

References

Beauchamp, T.L. and Childress, J.F. (1989) *Principles of Biomedical Ethics*, third edition. New York/Oxford: Oxford University Press.

Beddard, R. (1993) *Human Rights and Europe*, third edition. Cambridge: Grotius Publications.

Bolam v. Friern Hospital Management Committee QBD (1957) 2 *All ER*, 118.

Bulletin of Medical Ethics (1988a) **40**, July.

Bulletin of Medical Ethics (1988b) **44**, November, 18–22.

Bulletin of Medical Ethics (1992a) **75**, February, 3–4.

Bulletin of Medical Ethics (1992b) **76**, March, 8–10.

Crawford v. Charing Cross Hospital (1953) *The Times*, 8 December.

Department of Health (1991) *Local Research Ethics Committees, NHS Executive Guidelines*. HSG(91)5.

Department of Health (1994) *Consultation Paper on Confidentiality*, 10 August.

Editorial (1986) *Bulletin of Medical Ethics*, **12**, March, 1.

F v. West Berkshire HA (1989) 2 *Weekly Law Report*, 1025; 2 *All England Reports*, 545.

Gillick v. West Norfolk and Wisbech AHA and the DHSS (1985) 3 *All England Reports*, 402.

Law Commission (1991, 1993) *Law Commission Consultation Paper* 119 (1991) and 128, 129 and 130 (1993). HMSO.

Pearson Report (1978) Royal Commission on Civil Liberty and Compensation for Personal Injury, Cmnd 7054. London: HMSO.

R v. Brown and others (1993) *House of Lords Times Law Report*, 12 March.

Re C (adult: refusal of medical treatment) (1994) 1 *All England Reports*, 819.

Re W (also known as Re J) (a minor) (child in care: medical treatment) (1992) 3 *Weekly Law Report*, 758 CA.

RCN (1993) *Ethics Related to Research in Nursing*, revised.

Sidaway v. Board of Governors of Royal Bethlem and Maudsley Hospital (1985) 2 *Weekly Law Report*, 480.

The Times (1993) Andrew Pierce Cancer Centre threatens to sue over critical report. 8 November.

10

Philosophical Aspects

Louise de Raeve

> ... nursing is essentially a practice-based discipline and thus the purpose of nursing research should not be, as Field and Morse and many others claim, to develop nursing knowledge, but to develop nursing *practice* (Rolfe, 1994, p. 970).

The above remark by Rolfe suggests that a shift of emphasis is appearing in nursing research in response to a continuous concern about the "theory–practice gap". This concern raises questions about both the dissemination and relevance of research, but it is worth noting that this does not seem to be a preoccupation of nursing alone. Guba and Lincoln (1989) make reference to similar difficulties in the field of education research.

That there is a "theory–practice gap" is as common a refrain in nursing discourse as "nursing is a research-based profession", although the latter seems more expressive of intention than reality. Nevertheless, there has certainly been a rapid growth of interest in and practice of nursing research since the 1960s. In relation to this, therefore, it seems somewhat dispiriting that much of this new effort still appears to have relatively little impact on practice. The question one is compelled to ask is "Why?"

Clearly, part of the difficulty has been that in the process of developing new expertise, some nursing research has been of rather poor quality, and one might be relieved that work of this kind has not had much impact. Another contributing factor would be the difficulty that good nurse-researchers have in obtaining adequate funding to do work on a sufficiently large scale to have the impact that might be desired. However, these factors and doubtless many others are not in my view central to the difficulty. As nurses, I think we need to ask two fundamental questions:

(1) What are nurse-researchers trying to achieve?
(2) Is it achievable?

In response to the first question, it seems to me that nursing research has two central aims. One concerns the identity of nursing: we want to know what nursing is; and the other concerns the wish to promote good nursing care and to understand failures of practice with the aim of rectifying the situation. Obviously these two approaches are connected conceptually, for if one does not know the nature of an activity such as nursing, one can hardly be said to be in a position to evaluate with much insight, good or bad instances of it. Being able to evaluate a complex activity such as nursing is part and parcel of what "knowing how to nurse" means. In addition, nurses nurse people which means that any evaluation of nursing will include a moral dimension. Combined with the technologies and skills required for care, nursing is an inherently moral activity where certain moral attitudes are considered necessary for the delivery of good care. Professional ideologies on this matter may reflect different moral values in different cultures (Minami, 1985) and at different historical periods within any one culture (Winslow, 1984).

It is perhaps significant that if I reflect upon nursing research of the 1970s, the names that spring to mind are of people such as Felicity Stockwell (1972) for the work she and others did by carefully examining instances of the practice of nursing and providing the profession with some very uncomfortable illustrations of bad practice. However, in the last decade or so, I think it is true to say that nursing has become increasingly preoccupied with its own identity and this seems to have promoted a form of research which rather than purely examining dimensions of good and bad care has tried to capture and formulate the essence of nursing. The search for this seems to be driven by the somewhat elusive carrot of professional status (equal to but different from medicine) and by an increasing concern that in a climate of dwindling resources in health care, professional nursing may largely disappear in favour of care assistants, unless a convincing account can be given of what professional nursing is and why it might be important to preserve such a function.

Hopes have therefore been attached to the idea that a universal theory or at least a model of nursing could be produced such that from then onwards it would simply be a question of refining the work. Unfortunately, this approach has not borne the expected fruit, for while many descriptive and insightful accounts as to the true nature of nursing were put forward, there was a proliferation of competing views rather than any emerging uniformity. Individual nurses had their preferences but the criteria used for deciding between these accounts was not standardised and thus tended to reflect some amalgamation of the personal values and professional experience of individuals.

Despair at this picture led to another vision which questioned the whole approach. Theories and models had been invented rather than developed empirically and what was now needed was meticulous documentation of what nurses in fact did and of how they thought about their work, to generate "bottom up" rather than "top down" theory. At this point, nurse theorists turned to the research methods in vogue at the time, to help them. Grounded Theory (Glaser and Strauss, 1968), with its claim to be well grounded in reality, was one obvious candidate.

While not in the least wanting to deny the value of such an approach, I do want to question some of its fundamental aims. Firstly, the approach assumes that the question "what is the nature of nursing?" can be given a universal answer and that the problem is simply to do sufficient work to get there. Secondly, it is questionable whether grounded theory could ever generate the sort of theory nurses asking the first question were hoping for.

Rejection of a Universal Account of Nursing

In 1990, Cash wrote an interesting article about this question and stated:

> If the argument that I am going to present [is true], that nursing is not a unitary concept, that crudely, nursing is what nursing does, then the current problems in the definition of nursing or the attempted reduction to the concepts of, for example, caring or adaptation is theoretically misguided (Cash, 1990, p. 249).

This argument Cash pursues by showing that whatever one may single out as the essence of nursing, e.g. "care" or "the promotion of self-care", one merely ends up demonstrating that it is a necessary but not a sufficient condition for nursing. In other words, ideas of "care" or "self-care" are equally features of other professions such as occupational therapy and social work. Cash further suggests that when different branches of nursing are compared, e.g. surgical nursing and health visiting, some relationship can be found, but it is not clear that these are "exclusively nursing relationships" (Cash, 1990, p. 253). In addition, the surgical nurse might in fact have more in common with the surgical houseman and the health visitor with the social worker, than these two branches of nursing have with each other.

The picture that Cash offers instead is to see the various types and kinds of nursing as related through a series of "family resemblances". This is an idea that he has taken from Wittgenstein (1968, paragraph 67) and Bambrough (1960–61). Wittgenstein addresses the question of what is a game and wonders what might be said to be the feature or features that all games (e.g. board-games, card-games, ball-games, Olympic games, etc.) have in common (paragraph 66). He notes that some features that some games share, e.g. being "amusing" or having "winners and losers" are not consistent for all games, and he concludes that there are no universally shared features which would enable one to say "This . . . is what a game is." Wittgenstein says that instead:

> we see a complicated network of similarities overlapping and criss-crossing: sometimes overall similarities, sometimes similarities of detail (Wittgenstein, 1968, paragraph 66).

He goes on to call these "family resemblances" because

> the various resemblances between members of a family: build, features, colour of eyes, gait, temperament, etc. etc. overlap and criss-cross in the same way (Wittgenstein, 1968, paragraph 67).

Cash (1990) suggests that it would be fruitful to see nursing as a similar sort of concept. With reference to games, Wittgenstein observes that our inability to say what a game is in general and our reliance on describing or demonstrating particular games to answer the question "what is a game?" is not an expression of our ignorance. He says "we do not know the boundaries [of the concept] because none have been drawn" (paragraph 69), but this does not render the concept unusable. He also says that we can draw a boundary for a special purpose, and of course nursing does this all the time when considering whether a new initiative taken by a nurse is properly an extended role of nursing or simply not nursing at all. We know from our professional history that there is nothing permanently fixed about these boundaries.

Cash's conclusion seems to be that it might be liberating to think of nursing in this way because energies could be focused more profitably on trying to understand the nature of particular branches of nursing and we may find then that much of the doubt disappears. Perhaps we already know quite well what health visiting, surgical nursing, medical nursing, psychiatric nursing, etc. are.

Can Grounded Theory Meet Nurses' Expectations?

Maintaining the assumption for the purposes of argument that asking: "what is nursing?" is a coherent question, then the issue becomes: Can grounded theory generate "theory from data" (Glaser and Strauss, 1968, p. 1) in a way which will help this enterprise? My contention is that more may be being claimed for the method than it is in fact able to deliver.

Glaser and Strauss make it perfectly clear that their inductive method of research is in reaction to the previous dominance of grand theories in sociology such as those of Durkheim. They state:

> In contrasting grounded theory with logico-deductive theory and discussing and assessing their relative merits in ability to fit and work (predict, explain, and be relevant), we have taken the position that the adequacy of a theory of sociology today cannot be divorced from the process by which it is generated (Glaser and Strauss, 1968, p. 5).

However, while reacting against what went before, it seems to me that grounded theory also incorporates some assumptions that were possibly implicit within such grand theories. One such assumption seems to be the notion of what "data" are. Implicit within Glaser and Strauss's view is, I think, the idea that one can have confidence in the objectivity of data and thus the more one's theory is "grounded" in it, the more reliable and the truer therefore it will be. Glaser and Strauss do not believe that only one theory could emerge from the same data, nor that a good theory would not be subject to revision and perhaps eventual replacement, but their confidence in their method seems to be to do with a sense that a meticulously worked out theory done in accordance with their method will at least be more in touch with the real world than a theory construed from an armchair. It would be odd to suggest that there is not something in this, but all scientific methods are likely to have their limitations since they present "a way" of seeing the world, and thus one may need to be mindful of what these limitations are.

Clarke has something to say about one such limit when he observes:

> The point is that, to an uncertain degree, this is what is taking place in research: an assumption of meanings coming from a procedure which is "set" to regard words in a conceptually familiar way (Clarke, 1992, p. 247).

Clarke describes a little experiment to show what he means by presenting the same sentence to several people and asking them to identify the key ideas in it (a procedure required by grounded theory for the identification of codes and categories). Clarke's evidence suggested that different people may see rather different meanings, but that people from the same professional background have a reasonably consistent view. Nothing beyond speculation can be concluded from such a tiny study, but Clarke observes:

> Six of the subjects in this mini-study worked in a psychiatric institute permeated by a "counselling" and "sociality" language – especially the humanistic language represented by the work of, for example, Rogers (1970) – the word "acceptance" [which had appeared in the original sentence] might contain an enticement quality which outranks the (otherwise) familiar words in the sentence . . . (Clarke, 1992, p. 246).

Clarke's suggestion can, however, be quite well supported philosophically. Consider the language we usually use about things, e.g. "that's a table", "it's a comfortable chair", etc., and the language we use about people, e.g.

- "The treatment has a 50% chance of failure."
- "That scar must have been a nasty wound."
- "Removing her feeding tube killed her."

The point is that in the case of the language of things, objects may have no inherent value associated with them, although I can attach value by speaking of a "comfortable chair". Such language is quite different in this respect from the language used to speak about the behaviour of people towards each other.

All of the above examples can be restated differently, e.g.

- "The treatment has a 50% chance of success."
- "That scar is a tribal mark."
- "Removing her feeding tube enabled her to die."

In each of these three cases, the fact of treatment with a certain percentage outcome, the fact of a scar and the fact of removing a feeding tube are described; in the former illustration they were evaluated negatively and in the latter positively. Furthermore, while I can talk about chairs without having to introduce any question of their value (I may simply want to count them) I can't speak of removing a feeding tube without being committed to an evaluation of what was done. I cannot give a neutral description of the event at all. At this point someone might claim that saying: "Her feeding tube was removed thus causing her death" is a neutral account but, in reply, I would say that this description is morally ambiguous, not neutral and that it would never be read neutrally since the context of the remark and further details would quickly make the utterer's moral views clear and the reader's own moral attitude would inform how the described event was interpreted.

Here, someone could say that in my earlier example of counting chairs, since ordinarily we do not count chairs for no purpose, the context would make it clear why I needed to count them. This surely introduces value too (although not moral value). In reply, I would claim that this is contingently true (i.e. it could be otherwise), not necessarily true beyond the obvious (and weak idea) that any objects in the world that are named or created must have some significance and thus general value, in our lives. This weak idea of value is not nearly strong enough to capture what is at stake when we talk about what we do to each other as human beings.

Hence one can see that treating social data as if they were to be captured objectively in the way we talk about things is perhaps a rather ill-conceived idea which may lead to confusion. What counts as social data may be construed from different perspectives which reflect different social interests and activities and when such data are described, it is extremely unlikely, if not impossible, that any such description can be presented in value neutral terms. Moreover, where the phenomena being studied are human beings and their reactions to each other, these evaluations will frequently have a moral component.

What the nurse-researcher sees as data, a psychologist or sociologist may not, although both might have the same typed transcript of the interview in front of them. This is one of the reasons why I suspect Glaser and Strauss are absolutely right when they claim:

> One property of an applied grounded theory must be clearly understood: the theory can be developed only by professionally trained sociologists, but can be applied by either laymen or sociologists (Glaser and Strauss, 1968, p. 249).

By using the method in nursing as nurse-researchers, we seem to think that we will thereby be developing nursing theory, from scratch. This notion is somewhat at odds with the view that data, however meticulously described and categorised, cannot spontaneously generate any theory without someone's vision that sees the relationships and significances this way rather than that. Seeing likely construals of relationships will depend on the researcher's sensitivity to the data but it will not be divorced from a background of understanding of the theoretical constructions that underpin one's discipline. Evans Pritchard impresses Glaser and Strauss (1968, p. 148) for making no reference in his monogram to current theories of magic and witchcraft. Nevertheless, they assume that he was thoroughly familiar with them but chose to try and take a fresh look, which led to the development of his own highly original formulation. However, Evans Pritchard could not have done this without some reference to his professional background or he would have been in danger of seeing nothing of any great sociological interest at all. "Perceivers without concepts . . . are blind" (MacIntyre, 1985, p. 79).

Sociology and anthropology are academic disciplines which survive through being appropriately dependent upon the traditions and activities of groups, cultures and sub-cultures. Their business is to glean data and construct theoretical explanations and formulations of such behaviours. Such explanations clearly have potential use to the groups studied and/or to the wider society within which they occur and to the social group(s) that for benign or exploitative reasons choose to promote such studies.

Nursing, however, is quite different. It is an activity which provides a service to people in need. It is not primarily an academic discipline, since its primary focus is not research and the generation of theory (unlike sociology, history, physics, etc.) One might therefore wonder how it was thought that nursing could generate theory from data from the apparent position of a theoretical vacuum (not knowing what nursing really is). As I understand it, this is precisely the point that Robyn Holden (1991) makes in her criticism of the phenomenological nature of much nursing research. She says:

> Simply providing a description of events is, in my view, one of the major shortcomings of phenomenology . . . If phenomenology has no point of reference beyond description one is tempted to exclaim "So What?" (Holden, 1991, p. 390).

She suggests that there has to be a

> theoretical framework within which the psychological significance of the patient's utterances can be understood, and from which the uniting principles underscoring the patient's utterances can be derived (Holden, 1991, p. 389).

Holden's personal preference is for psychoanalytic theory but it is the idea of any "well-conceived psychological theory" that she wishes to promote. In addition of course, there is no reason to think that, given relevant contexts, sociological and anthropological perspectives might not be equally useful to nursing. The point is that rather than nurses looking for nursing theory *per se*, time might be better spent trying to use existing theories in psychology and sociology to understand better the interactive processes in nursing that many nurse-researchers so carefully describe.

Who might be best equipped to do this? It seems to me that it might be those nurses who are extremely competent researchers and who have a sophisticated understanding of a relevant theoretical discipline such as psychology or sociology and of the different schools of thought that exist within them or, alternatively, those social scientists (such as Judith Lathlean) who develop an abiding interest in nursing. The multiple analysis of nursing from several different theoretical perspectives might be stimulating and enriching to the profession and help to promote new insights into patient care. However, very few nurses will either want or be able to operate at this level. Is there no scope for any other kind of nursing research?

At the beginning of this chapter, I quoted from Rolfe's (1994) article and made a distinction between nursing research being concerned with establishing the identity of nursing and its being concerned with questions of good and bad practice. Perhaps as Rolfe suggests, we should be less preoccupied with developing nursing knowledge and more concerned with improving our practice. This way our knowledge of nursing is likely to grow spontaneously. Such a process is nicely exemplified in the following description from neonatal nursing concerning babies withdrawing from crack cocaine:

> We've trained nurses to evaluate babies using scoring sheets so there's not so much guess work involved or so much opinion of, "Well, I think this is really a fussy baby; therefore it must be withdrawing" (Tanner *et al.*, 1993, p. 279).

The commentary continues:

> The distinction between fussiness associated with withdrawal and fussiness associated with other causes is learned over time by learning the patterns of particular babies who are later confirmed to actually be withdrawing from crack cocaine and contrasting that knowledge of these "crack babies" with others who are fussy for other reasons and who have different patterns of fussiness. Thus, knowing particular babies sets up the possibility of knowing a patient population by collecting instances and contrasts over time. And in turn, knowing a patient population sets up a context for knowing variations and particularity within that population (Tanner *et al.*, 1993, p. 279).

The question therefore arises as to the best way of promoting good nursing practice, of understanding the competing visions that may constitute this and of describing and understanding nursing failures such that remedial action becomes possible. Nursing research may be accomplished in describing the contrast between overt nursing values and those which seem implicit in practice and it may be good at describing practice as it is but its capacity to effect change and its relevance to the contexts studied often seems poor. This is in part an issue of dissemination, but of course if the problem of relevance were to be thoroughly addressed, the problem of dissemination might disappear.

The difficulty seems to be how to pursue research that is considered relevant by practitioners and not just researchers and then how to present the findings in such a way that even unpalatable truths can be integrated in some constructive way without those studied being paralysed yet further by increasing guilt and demoralisation. Clearly one has to combine criticism with some constructive and realistic suggestions for change. To engage in this process may require understanding resistance to change for all the reasons that Menzies Lyth (1988) described decades ago.

Nolan and Grant (1993) suggest that what is required is an action research type of framework which designs research questions around practitioner's needs and builds into the research a process of change. Such an idea is further endorsed by Rolfe (1994). This extended idea of action research, which combines research with quality assurance and change theory, can incorporate within it any kind of research method, as judged appropriate for the particular question in hand. It is interesting that while not purporting to be action research in any traditional sense, Roger Watson's research project (described in Chapter 1) might fit the extended notion of the concept rather well, despite the fact that the method used was experimental.

The traditional action research approach (as described by Lathlean in Chapter 3) has a clear collaborative framework and would appear to fit well with the cooperative inquiry group structure promoted by Reason (1988). Nevertheless, the traditional descriptions of action research (Rapoport, 1970; Susman and Evered, 1978) make it clear that it is seen as being a social science method and one which contributes to the theoretical knowledge of this discipline as well as helping to solve organisational problems. The collaborative idea also has some potential limits for according to Rapoport the researcher maintains a degree of control: "The problem presented by the client was taken as data but not as mandate" (Rapoport, 1970, p. 502). This means that in promoting a more general conception of action research, its nature may be being subtly changed which is why it may be preferable to speak of an extended conception and a traditional conception of this research approach.

The cooperative inquiry group structure (Reason, 1988) may be of particular use in nursing since those areas of nursing practice where care is often particularly poor (e.g. psychogeriatric care) may be the very last to perceive a need for research, out of a combination of perhaps guilt and a disbelief that anything could change for the better. There is thus a problem of initiating sufficient interest for a research enterprise to be owned, to some extent at least, by the group to be researched upon/with. Setting up a cooperative inquiry group might be an interesting way of embarking and of course there is no reason why such a group could not involve patient representatives from community health councils or relevant self-help groups.

However, in keenness to promote these kinds of ideas, one should perhaps not lose sight of just how complex the combined role of researcher and change agent actually is. Judith Lathlean (Chapter 3) has described the difficulties she faced in trying to say what needs to be said in a way that is honest, without it being experienced as critical to the extent that people simply reject the ideas. It was for good reasons that Rapoport (1970, p. 503) elected to divide the activities so that he did the research work and a colleague with sophisticated therapeutic skills helped present the findings and interpretations. Peter Reason (1988, p. 31) also refers to the idea of dividing the functions between an inquiry process facilitator and a group process facilitator. Few nurses would currently have these dual skills, but perhaps we should be training those who have a pervading interest in research to develop them.

Conclusion

This chapter has suggested that a research preoccupation with trying to work out the nature of nursing in general may not be a fruitful avenue of inquiry. It is argued that this is because (a) there may be no essence of nursing and (b) because even if there were, the research methods chosen are unlikely to be able to generate theory in a vacuum. It may thus be much more productive to examine different specialisms in nursing from different theoretical perspectives. This would demand of nurse-researchers that they acquire expertise in both research methods and in an explanatory academic discipline. It is envisaged that only a few nurses would have the interest and background for this sort of work. In addition, it has been suggested that a rather different and important line of research inquiry for nursing to undertake is the technical and moral investigation of nursing practice. Much work has already been done in this area, but the recommendation here is that greater emphasis be given to it. This would address issues such as the perceived shortfall between nursing ideals and actual practice in particular contexts and seek to interpret such information (drawing upon the more theoretical research previously described) in order to facilitate change. Bridging the theory–practice gap may require research to be more directly relevant to practitioners. To this end it has been suggested that nurse-researchers embrace an extended action research type of focus which, while not excluding the use of any relevant research method to obtain necessary data would aim to research in some degree of partnership with clinical nurses and patients.

References

Bambrough, R. (1960–61) Universals and family resemblances. *Proceedings of the Aristotelian Society*, **LXI**, 207–222.

Cash, K. (1990) Nursing models and the idea of nursing. *International Journal of Nursing Studies*, **27**(3), 249–256.

Clarke, L. (1992) Qualitative research: meaning and language. *Journal of Advanced Nursing*, **17**, 243–252.

Glaser, B. and Strauss, A. (1968) *The Discovery of Grounded Theory: Strategies for Qualitative Research*. London: Weidenfeld and Nicolson.

Guba, E.G. and Lincoln, Y.S. (1989) *Fourth Generation Evaluation*. Newbury Park, California: Sage Publications.

Holden, R.J. (1991) On applying psychoanalytic explanations in phenomenological research. *International Journal of Nursing Studies*, **28**(4), 387–396.

MacIntyre, A. (1985) *After Virtue*, second edition. London: Duckworth and Co. Ltd.

Menzies Lyth, I. (1988) *Containing Anxiety in Institutions*. London: Free Association Books.

Minami, H. (1985) East meets west: some ethical considerations. *International Journal of Nursing Studies*, **22**(4), 311–318.

Nolan, M. and Grant, G. (1993) Action research and quality of care: a mechanism for agreeing basic values as a precursor to change. *Journal of Advanced Nursing*, **18**, 305–311.

Rapoport, R.N. (1970) Three dilemmas in action research. *Human Relations*, **23**(6), 499–513.

Reason, P. (ed.) (1988) *Human Inquiry in Action*. London: Sage Publications.

Rolfe, G. (1994) Towards a new model of nursing research. *Journal of Advanced Nursing*, **19**, 969–975.

Stockwell, F. (1972) *The Unpopular Patient*. London: Royal College of Nursing.

Susman, G.I. and Evered, R.D. (1978) An assessment of the scientific merits of action research. *Administrative Science Quarterly*, **23**, 582–603.

Tanner, C.A., Benner, P., Chesla, C. and Gordon, D.R. (1993) The phenomenology of knowing the patient. *Image: Journal of Nursing Scholarship*, **25**(4), 273–280.

Winslow, G.R. (1984) From loyalty to advocacy: a new metaphor for nursing. *The Hastings Center Report*, June, 32–40.

Wittgenstein, L. (1968) *Philosophical Investigations* (translated by G. E. M. Anscombe). Oxford: Basil Blackwell.

III

Broader Issues

11

Ethical Review of Nursing Research

Neil Pickering

The subject of this chapter is ethical review of research; that is, the process, usually carried out by a committee, of (ideally) independent review of research protocols involving the use of human subjects.

In the course of this chapter, a number of specific questions will be taken up. In the first section, "Why have we got ethical review?" The second section considers a broader question, "What ways have been tried to carry it out?" A brace of questions are considered in the third section, concerning the current system in the UK: "What problems does the current UK system have in general?" and "What problems does the UK system have vis à vis nursing research in particular?" The fourth section considers "How are research ethics committees perceived by nurse-researchers?" The fifth section asks "What alternatives to the present system might be considered?"

A further, more general, question might also be borne in mind throughout. What is the nature of a review which claims to be *ethical*? From the first, it will be assumed that research on human subjects involves the use of a human being in a manner determined by science (of whatever sort). It is this which makes all such research morally sensitive. As is amply demonstrated in the earlier chapters of this book, such moral sensitivity is not confined to the stage of ethical review. The sensitive researcher may be faced with moral issues throughout a research project. But, at some point in the process of designing, developing and finally putting into practice a research protocol, the considerations of someone or body, as far as possible genuinely independent of the research, is morally obligatory. It will be suggested that there may be an intractable element to moral differences between morally sensitive individuals who have different roles with respect to a research protocol. This means that there is no guarantee that a nurse who proposes research and an ethics committee which reviews it, can be brought to see the protocol in the same light.

Why Have We Got Ethical Review of Human Subjects Research?

Some origins of concern

At the time of writing, the 50th anniversary commemorations of the liberation of Auschwitz have been going on around the world. Auschwitz was one place where Nazi doctors carried out "experiments" on the captive inmates. The horror of finding that doctors had carried out such experiments prompted the writing of the Nuremberg Code (Nuremberg Military Tribunals, 1949). Later came the Declaration of Helsinki and its subsequent revisions (see Appendix). Someone might say that the Nazi atrocities are an unusually gross perversion of the doctor's role, and the horror they provoked is to that extent uniquely appropriate to that example. Something of the same revulsion, however, may attach to other examples of the untrammelled use of human beings for experimental purposes.

The Tuskegee Syphilis study in the USA started before the Second World War and ended only in the 1970s. It set out to discover the natural history of syphilis, but was carried on long after the disease was curable by penicillin. The so-called science of the study, it might be said, had dictated that the sufferers remain untreated. The ultimate reaction to the study illustrates a general concern about research involving human subjects – simply, that what is (claimed as) scientifically correct and necessary may involve quite unacceptable harm to and treatment of the research subjects, and that this is true of all such research.

Historically, there were some noises in the UK at about the time the USA began to become seriously concerned (Royal College of Physicians, 1967, 1973; Department of Health and Social Security, 1975). Contemporary documents mention using committees to ensure that research is carried out ethically. The research ethics committee (REC) is one of the primary means to the end of ensuring that research on human subjects does not repeat (in however small a way) the horrors of the past.

But as late as 1988, when Paul Byrne compared the US and UK systems of ethical review, his comparison was somewhat to the disadvantage of the UK system at that time (Byrne, 1988). Byrne notes in his article how RECs in the UK had failed in some important instances, and he mentions in particular the case of Mrs Wigley, analysed also in Carolyn Faulder's book *Whose Body Is It?* (Faulder, 1985). In this case, which had taken place in 1981, RECs had allowed research to proceed knowing that no consent would be asked for. Mrs Wigley died in the course of the clinical trial, into which she was entered without her knowledge. At the time Byrne was writing, further worries had been raised by a report of the Institute of Medical Ethics into the review committee system in the UK (Nicholson, 1986).

Nurses, in 1988, would have been researching under the Royal College of

Nursing's 1977 guidelines (Royal College of Nursing, 1977) which state:

> In most instances the approval of the appropriate ethics committee will be necessary, but in any case the researcher would be wise to seek advice on the ethical aspects of the study (p. 3).

But Byrne's point is perhaps that the presence of guidelines and of RECs is not a guarantee of protection of human subjects. His recommendation, that in order to ensure it worked the system in the UK be given legal backing, has not been taken up.

Mary Armstrong, also writing in 1988, in the wake of Faulder's book and the IME Survey results, notes that nursing is "an art and a science" (Armstrong, 1988, p. 17). She adds: "Nursing research poses the same sort of dilemmas as medical research" (Armstrong, 1988, p. 18) and strikes a note not dissimilar to Byrne when she hints that the existence of a system of review and its proper operation are two quite different matters.

> It does not appear that many of the committees are asked to look at research projects in nursing ... One wonders how many nurse researchers have submitted a proper protocol to an ethical committee ... (Armstrong, 1988, p. 18).

Practice, in short, may sometimes not match rhetoric, and a problem arises as to how to make sure that, as far as possible, it does.

The intentions of ethical review root documents

Though practice may sometimes not match rhetoric, it is still worthwhile reflecting on some of the documents which have expressed the ideals of ethical review. Versions, particularly of the Declaration of Helsinki, may also have had an impact on the development of systems of ethical review of research (Bergkamp, 1988; Holm, 1992).

Among the "basic principles" of the Declaration of Helsinki (see Appendix) is the idea that "each experimental procedure involving human subjects should be clearly formulated in an experimental protocol which should be transmitted for consideration, comment and guidance to a specially appointed committee independent of the investigator and the sponsor" (p. 184). The primary consideration of this committee is to be that "in research on man, the interest of science and society should never take precedence over considerations related to the wellbeing of the subject" (p. 186).

Not taking precedence would not be the same as not being considered. Levine (1986) quotes the National Commission for the Protection of Human Subjects of Biomedical and Behavioral Research:

> ... the ethical conduct of research involving human subjects requires a balancing of society's interests in protecting the rights of subjects and in developing

knowledge that can benefit the subjects or society as a whole . . . (National Commission, 1978, pp. 1–2).

The nature of ethical review, if the National Commission *Report* is right, is that it requires a balancing of interests, rights, risks and harms.

Forms of Ethical Review

By form of ethical review is intended its institutional set up, its processes, procedures and other arrangements. Features of the UK system will first be described, and then features of two other systems (those of the USA and of Denmark).

The UK system

The UK system is in theory that established by the Department of Health guidelines *Local Research Ethics Committees* (Department of Health, 1991). In what follows, a number of its features will be drawn out, and some brief comment made upon them. (The numbers in brackets refer to the paragraphs in the Department's guidelines.)

(1) It is local review. The system is based upon the existing District Health Authorities (DHAs) (2.1). In addition, there are some central committees, attached, for instance, to some of the Royal Colleges, for instance the Royal College of General Practitioners (Drury, 1992) and there are a number of other RECs, some attached to the drug industry. The Local Research Ethics Committee (LREC) is responsible for reviewing research which will take place in the district (1.5).

(2) It is committee review. In this it follows the Helsinki Declaration. The Department recommendation is for between 8 and 12 members (2.4).

(3) It is DHA based, but is not an arm of management (1.1; 2.2). The committee exists to advise NHS bodies, which have the responsibility for making the final decision (1.1). But the committee is not a part of the DHA's management of health services, and so should be free from particular policies the DHA may have regarding research, resourcing and so on.

(4) Its role is to advise any (though not only) NHS bodies involved in human subjects research (1.1). Hence bodies not managed by the DHA may seek the advice of the committee, and this will include the NHS Hospital Trusts (1.2) and Family Health Service Authorities (1.2).

(5) Membership is supposed to include a lay element of at least two (2.5), and nurse membership is advised (2.5), in addition to medical professionals. A gender and age mix is also advised (2.5).

(6) Members are not generally paid for being on an LREC, and nor are researchers generally charged for using it. Secretarial and administrative support is provided by the DHA, and travel expenses are usually available to members.

(7) All research going on in NHS premises or on NHS patients or on their records is supposed to go to the LREC for approval (1.3). This point is affirmed in the RCN's *Ethics Related to Research in Nursing* (RCN Nursing Research Advisory Group, 1993, p. 11) and also in the nursing research Taskforce *Report* (Taskforce, 1993, p. 28). However, not all research on humans is expected to go to an LREC. For instance, Phase 1 drug trials involve no patients, and take place usually in special research units; but such protocols will go to independent committees within the industry. Nevertheless, the Department guidelines (Department of Health, 1991) urge researchers not otherwise falling under the guidelines to use the LREC and for these services the LREC may charge (2.17).

(8) There is no national committee in the UK, though the suggestion that one be formed has been floated (Benster and Pollock, 1992).

(9) The system in general bears no legal teeth. It is a form of self-regulation. One exception is research involving living human embryos and foetuses, which is restricted by law, and is, where allowed, permitted only under licence of the Human Fertilisation and Embryology Authority (Evans *et al.*, 1992, 6–34). However, two other reports left some responsibility for decisions concerning controversial areas of research in the hands of LRECs (Evans *et al.*, 1992, 6-35-7, 6-37-9; Department of Health, 1991, 1.3). These were the Polkinghorn and Clothier Committee Reports, the first into the use of foetuses and foetal material (Polkinghorn Committee, 1989), and the second into gene therapy (Clothier Committee, 1992).

The Government's obligation to bring into domestic law European Commission Directive 91/507/EEC amending 75/318/EEC has been fulfilled (Medicines Control Agency, 1995). It has been claimed that this, in effect, makes the latest version of the Declaration of Helsinki part of domestic law, and gives to the current LREC system a statutory basis (see, e.g., Evans *et al.*, 1992, 6–4). But the Declaration is referred to in the guidelines on Good Clinical Practice, and these remain guidelines, and not themselves part of the law. LRECs have three recourses if researchers ignore their decisions, or circumvent the system. The first is to report to the DHA, the second to report to any other NHS body involved, and the third to report the researcher to his or her professional body (3.22).

(10) The review is intended to be independent (1.1). The independence of the committees is supposed to be secured, first, by their not being an arm of DHA management, and not beholden, either, to any other NHS or non-NHS body (2.2); second, by their having a mixture of lay and health-care professional membership (2.4); third, by the withdrawal of

members for discussion of protocols in which they may have an interest (3.23); fourth, by their meeting in private, enabling members to express freely all their concerns (2.15); and fifth by members acting as free agents, and not as the representatives of their professional or other interests (2.6).

(11) With respect to accountability, public information relating to the work of particular LRECs currently amounts to their making annual reports (2.16). Minutes, for instance, are not publicised (2.15). There are two leading possibilities whereby LRECs or their members might find themselves being called to account in the courts, though neither is very likely to succeed. The first would relate to charges of negligence, against either individual members or the whole committee, and might come about if a research subject were to be harmed in the course of research, and the subject could show that the LREC had failed properly to review the protocol, for instance by failing to take expert advice in an area they knew themselves to be ignorant. Opinion seems to be that such charges would be very unlikely to succeed against individual members, or against the committee as a whole (Evans et al., 1992, 6–10) (2.11). The second possibility would arise in respect of the way a committee discharges its duty to reach its decisions (2.12), if members had undeclared personal interests in a particular protocol, or judged a protocol in an unreasonably biased way. The criterion of reasonability would be set by the way LRECs in general reached decisions (Evans et al., 1992, 6–10).

(12) There is no appeal from an LREC decision, except to take research elsewhere, or simply ignore the committee's verdict.

International comparisons

USA

The US system has come into being, gradually, since about 1967 (Byrne, 1988). At that time, a number of cases came to very public attention, of which the most notorious were the Tuskegee Syphilis study (mentioned earlier), and the Jewish Chronic Diseases Hospital study (Bergkamp, 1988). In an article published in the *New England Journal of Medicine* (Beecher, 1966) H. K. Beecher identified many more. A National Research Act came in 1974 (Department of Health Education and Welfare, 1974), followed by Commissions of Enquiry (National Commission, 1978) and then Federal regulations, the most recent being in 1981 (Department of Health and Human Services, 1981).

The current situation is that all human subjects research conducted or funded by the Department of Health and Human Services, or regulated by the Food and Drugs Administration must have the approval of an Institutional Review Board (IRB) before it can proceed. IRBs work under regulations of these departments. The regulations cover the membership of the Boards, their responsibilities and workings. An IRB is a body designated by an institution (for instance, a nursing college such as the Yale University School of Nursing, but institution is widely defined in the regulations) to protect the rights of human research subjects. These federal regulations were extended in 1981 to all federally funded research, whether taking place in "institutions" or not (Levine, 1986, p. 325; Herman, 1989, p. 2). Thus review boards, sometimes known as Non-Institutional Review Boards, work under the same guidelines (Herman, 1989).

Denmark

Søren Holm (Holm, 1992) notes three features of the Danish system which (he claims) contrast with both US and UK systems. First, Danish RECs are independent of specific institutions, being established on a geographical basis. Second, Danish RECs are comparatively small (six to ten members), but have, by law, a comparatively high proportion of lay members (from 1992, parity plus 1) and must have a gender balance. Third, in addition to the RECs there is a central national committee. The role of this committee is interesting as it provides, among other things, a court of appeal against an REC decision. The membership of the central committee is balanced like that of the RECs, but it is much larger than the local committees, being made up of two representatives from each REC.

Initially, Holm notes, the system was founded upon the Declaration of Helsinki, and had no legal teeth. In this, it was much like the British system is now. Research generally went through the system because publishing and funding research that did not tended to be more difficult, and there was always the danger of "exposure". In 1992 the system was given a statutory basis. This statute has a section giving the ethical principles upon which the system is based, and Holm describes this as more or less a translation of the Helsinki document (Holm, 1992, p. 9). Failure to comply with committee decisions is now a criminal offence.

Difficulties with the UK System

Considered in this section are difficulties with the system which may affect nurse-researchers. Some of the problems have wider implications too.

Multicentre research

Multicentre research involves human research subjects in multiple locations, though the precise number of locations that make a trial multicentre is not defined (Evans, 1992a, p. 12). Nursing research may well be multicentre. If the research is to be carried out in many locations, then many different LRECs may be entitled to look at the protocol. This can cause problems for the researcher. For instance, one committee may request changes to the protocol, when other committees may approve of it as it is, and still others suggest different changes. Some committees may reject the proposed research, while others accept it, which may leave the researcher in a quandary. Each committee may (and perhaps should) request to meet the person or persons who will be carrying out the research, which could involve a researcher in much travelling. In short, the process of getting a multicentre research proposal through the ethical review system is likely to be longer and more complicated than getting a protocol through review by one committee only. But, LRECs have a responsibility locally which means they have individually a duty to review such protocols.

In 1992 (after their guidelines had been published ad hopefully put into effect) the Department of Health found that their suggestion, in the guidelines, that multicentre trials be ethically reviewed by one committee on behalf of hers (Department of Health, 1991, 2.18) had been found wanting, and some alternative was needed (Benster and Pollock, 1992; Pelerin and Hall, 1992; Moodie and Marshall, 1992 The report (Evans, 1992a) they commissioned described the existing review as prone to inefficiency and ineffectiveness.

The charge of inefficiency resulted from the time taken to respond to multicentre studies by some committees. In one extreme (non-nursing) case, up to two years had elapsed since the protocol had been sent, and no response had been forthcoming at all from some committees (Evans, 1992a, p. 13). The charge of ineffectiveness arose where variations in responses to protocols were perceived as being arbitrary by those trying to get the research ethically approved. It also arose where local committee members perceived that ethical review by a central committee lacked independence, yet felt pressure from central approval of the protocol to approve it likewise. Central committees that review multicentre protocols include the committee of the Royal College of GPs (Drury, 1992). Where the collaboration of such central committees with local committees was perceived as potentially useful, it was noted that full and appropriate communication was difficult to achieve. To meet these problems, the report (Evans, 1992a) recommended, among other things, the standardisation of practice (for instance in the use of pro formas), improved communications between central and local committees, improved expertise of review at the centre, better servicing of local committees, and greater opportunities for local committee members to meet and exchange ideas. The possible role of training for LREC members was also mentioned.

However, while training, and the other measures recommended by the report, might do something to reduce arbitrary variations in response to multicentre research, it is unlikely to remove all variation. Indeed, someone might say that to attempt to eradicate all variation is to mistake the nature of moral considerations in ethical review of human subjects research. Consider, for instance, the Department's own suggestion, that one local committee review a protocol on behalf of others. This sounds like the Danish system, discussed by Søren Holm (1992, p. 9). He implies that it is only where there is clear homogeneity within a particular society (as there is in Denmark) that committees can feel confident in leaving an important decision to one of their number. The confidence arises because the criteria which are applied by the committees tends to uniformity (Holm, 1992, p. 9).

Such uniformity may not exist in the UK, which has a far larger population, and considerable racial, religious and cultural diversity. But this is a matter of opinion; Robert Levine, citing the American rights-based approach, contrasted this with the UK, which he saw as generally cohesive and deferential in nature (Levine, 1988, p. 133).

Someone may also point out that, in moral matters, disagreements can be intractable, such that two people having divergent attitudes to the same protocol may be simply unable to agree on its merits. One may weigh the harm the protocol risks to the subjects as being less significant than the potential benefits of the research; another may disagree. Since, on this account, the "weighing" which is referred to here is not like the weighing which scales may do for someone, there is nothing which will prove that one person has weighed things rightly and the other wrongly. Indeed, these terms "rightly" and "wrongly" can have only a moral meaning here, i.e. they are expressions of judgement, not measurement.

Different kinds of protocol

LRECs are called upon to pass judgement on a wide variety of protocol types (Department of Health, 1991, 3.3). It may be that they will not be equally familiar with all those designs and methodologies that come before them. It could be argued that design and methodology are scientific matters, and are in virtue of this not the subject of ethical review. However, if a protocol's design is such that it cannot achieve its ends, then to carry out the proposed research is at the very least a waste of time, and hence of resources, and may constitute a risk to subjects without any hope of benefit to any patient. Waste and risk are moral notions, in this context, so scientifically bad research is a moral issue. If follows that the concerns of an ethics committee must extend to the design of a protocol. But, of course, it follows from this that failing to understand the science of a protocol is itself to fail fully ethically to review the research.

How might this affect review of nursing research? Armstrong argued, in 1988, that the LREC should be concerned that nursing research has a "proper protocol . . . methodology . . . and precautions" (Armstrong, 1988, p. 17) in just the same way as medical research proposals. Armstrong may have meant that legitimate nursing research would have to take on the same criteria for a scientifically good protocol as was appropriate for medical research. Historically, it is this medical model which RECs have tended to work with. Faced with this in the USA in 1980, Ada Jacox argued that nursing research had its own methodology, but that this was often misunderstood by the IRBs. She comments:

> When proposals are submitted that do not fall into the category of experimentally designed research and when they are focused primarily on the study of psychosocial behaviour the approval process often becomes extended and frequently the proposal is disapproved (Jacox, 1980, p. 62).

Nursing research studies health care, a different category from the "essentially biological view of illness" which "does not adequately take into account the interaction between biological and behavioral science that is needed in the study of health care" (Jacox, 1980, p. 62).

Here, at least implicitly, is the idea that the ethical review committees need to be educated themselves. If they are not, two problems may follow. First, the research may be judged on inappropriate criteria by those who are ignorant or dismissive of the criteria it does conform to. (For instance, a control group might be expected, and nursing protocols not having one might be rejected; or the research may not aim to test a hypothesis at all, and may be accounted faulty because of that.) As a result, potentially very beneficial nursing research might not get done, and non-beneficial practices might continue or more beneficial practices not be introduced.

Second, as Lützén implies in this volume, ignorance of how some nursing research protocols may develop after LREC approval may lead LRECs unfamiliar with such protocols too easily to approve them. For instance, the harmlessness of initial questions proposed in a questionnaire may hide how an interview may develop. Moreover, where there may be a hypothesis the protocol intends to test, that may be finalised only during the research, a committee which is unaware of this may fail to ask what the research might end up trying to find out.

The NHS reforms

In the year that the Department of Health published its guidelines directing DHAs to set up LRECs (Department of Health, 1991), the 1990 reforms of the NHS also came into effect. These may affect the DHAs, and hence the LREC system set up through them.

Two such effects may converge to reduce the number of DHAs, for instance. The first is the placing of purchasing power in GP Fundholding Practices, so that DHAs no longer are the sole purchasers of health care. The second is the fact that bargaining power is greater for larger purchasing organisations. Any reduction in the number of DHAs, resulting from amalgamations brought on by a combination of these two forces, will take place without any consonant reduction in the amount of research. A possible result of this is illustrated by the East London and City Health Authority, an amalgamation of three DHAs. The three LRECs were also amalgamated, meaning that all research of the relevant kind taking place in East London would need to come through the one committee (Doyal, 1994, p. 16).

Someone might suggest that Trust-based RECs may take on some of the work. The Department guidelines (Department of Health, 1991) do not rule out such RECs, but its guidance is clear that they cannot be used instead of LRECs. What might justify this position? The fear may be that a Trust may stand to benefit from some of the research it carries out, or that is carried out in its premises, or on its patients; and may stand to lose from other research. Bergkamp (1988), noting that both the Dutch and the USA systems involve institution-based ethical review, outlines concerns about the independence of their review being compromised by these institutional connections. However, Holm (1992, p. 9) argues that where there may be very distinct ethical outlooks in institutions (perhaps those with specific religious bases), a non-institutional form of review may be unacceptable.

Practical difficulties

The primary practical problem for some LRECs is the number of protocols they have to review. Concern has, implicitly, been expressed about how nursing research protocols may have added to this practical problem. For instance, a Welsh National Board advisory paper highlights two needs in connection with this. These are the needs, first, for proper peer review of nursing research before it gets to a (perhaps) overworked LREC; and second, for clarity as to when original research involving patients (and hence LREC review) is really necessary (Welsh National Board, 1991).

Also connected with LREC workload may be a point Lützén makes in this volume. Where the actual knowledge to be gained is not specifiable until the first results are in, and where, given these results, the protocol may change, the question arises as to whether an LREC should ask to see the protocol again in its developing forms. The Department of Health guidelines make clear that monitoring research protocols is to be carried out (Department of Health, 1991, 2.14) and most LRECs expect changes to protocols to be notified to them (major changes may require renewed review) and any serious adverse events may need to be reported to the committee. However, the extra burden of work close monitoring may give rise to may mean that it is not welcomed. Already, there is evidence that continued review of research is not everywhere a priority (Evans, 1992b, p. 20).

How the LREC May Be Perceived By Researchers

The gatekeeper

As with any human institution, the LREC may come to represent quite different things to different people. Ersser (Chapter 4) describes the LREC as one of a number of gatekeepers. Armstrong sees it in this way too, but for her the gate might be said to have a rather specific meaning. She notes that in 1988 "in some districts . . . a separate 'Nursing Ethics Research Committee' has been set up specifically to review nursing research" (Armstrong, 1988, p. 18). She insists, however, that nursing research goes through "the same scrutiny" ("gate") as medical research (p. 18). This may have something to do with its status as a "science . . . treated like any other science" (p. 17). That is, passing through the LREC is part of the process of scientific legitimation of nursing research. Another source of objection to separate ethical review of nursing research protocols is that it might cut off the possibility of increased understanding, in the wider research community, of what nursing research aims to achieve, and its methods.

However, another implicit conception of the LREC as gatekeeper is that it can be educated to allow through protocols with criteria of science different to those of medical research. If this is possible, then education roles have been posited for both researcher and reviewer. Is there, then, some hope that, in the end, they may be brought to see things more or less eye to eye?

Collaborative model

If some principle could be said to contain the idea that the relationship of nurse-researcher and the RECs approached should be collaborative, it is perhaps this: that good research is a vital part of what the NHS does. This is likely to be agreed by both committee members and researchers, and is the foremost assumption in the Department's guidelines (Department of Health, 1991, 1.1).

But, it may be argued, the nature of ethical review is such that such collaboration must have a limit. The notion of "independence" provides the source of this limit. Independence, taken in its strongest meaning, must imply independence not only from the research, but also of judgement about the researcher. This does not mean that the LREC *must* see the researcher in a bad light. It means, however, that the LREC must be free to reject the researcher's justifications for carrying out the research, and be free, if necessary, to question the competence of the researcher, or the adequacy of the facilities and/or time available to the researcher.

It will be noted, perhaps, that the grounds of this rejection might be that the envisaged advance in knowledge and benefit for patients is either illusory or is to be achieved at too high a price in terms of risk to the subjects of the proposed research. In either case, the appeal may be to principles (of good research and subject protection) which will probably be held by both researcher and committee. But, someone might argue, moral judgements in particular cases may differ even if moral principles are held in common.

Alternative Systems

Given the necessary potential limitation of collaboration between REC and researcher, the "gatekeeper" image seems to a degree appropriate. However, the present incumbent of the post of gatekeeper – the LREC constituted according to the DOH guidelines – could be replaced.

The mainly nurse REC

If currently constituted LRECs may use the wrong model of research to judge nursing research by, an alternative – committees which are made up of those most likely to understand it, and so give it a fair hearing – seems to have some justification. In addition, such committees could take from the LRECs the burden of reviewing potentially large numbers of nursing research protocols. One candidate for this role would be a committee made up mainly of nurses. Such a committee would have the advantages of being (or becoming) expert in nursing research, and, moreover, sensitive to the needs of patients. Lay representatives could be included, as on LRECs.

One argument against the institution of any such proposal would be this: any committee in which there is a dominance of one professional interest is unacceptable, particularly where the dominant profession is judging other members of itself. All nurses today know that their profession is asserting its own knowledge and research base. (It does not follow, of course, that they cannot be, or never are, sceptical about this.) In this atmosphere researcher and committee might be perceived to share too many professional goals and values. It will quickly be spotted that this same argument holds against any REC which is composed principally of members of one professional interest group (for instance, doctors) and which is charged with reviewing the research protocols of members of that same profession. (This is precisely the suspicion sometimes held by some LRECs of central review committees which are attached to particular Royal Colleges.)

It might be a little hasty to allow the proposal to lapse at that, however. Someone might argue in its favour that it is not clear that a mainly nurse committee will be easier on nursing research protocols submitted to it than any other committee. Rather, it might tend to extreme rigour, so as to divert any criticism, and maintain standards. However, in response, it may be said that the determination to be rigorous in one's review cannot replace actual professional independence from the protocol, the researcher, and all they stand for. On the other hand, the level of independence insisted upon here is greater than that insisted upon in the Department's guidelines, which asks only that members drawn from a variety of particular professions put professional interests aside in their consideration of research protocols.

The majority-lay REC

It may be argued that true independence of proposed research and proposing researcher comes from someone's personal and professional disinterestedness in the protocol. But, some interests are expected to be expressed by members of LRECs – the interests of the research subjects. Someone might say: if it is the interests of the subjects themselves that are paramount, then why not ask them, and make the asking of them the basis of ethical review of all human subjects research? Two practical alternatives (at least) may reflect these words.

The first, and perhaps more radical, alternative is that LRECs are allowed to veto research only for scientific reasons, leaving all judgements of value (chiefly ethical value) to the people most concerned, that is those who are asked to take part in the research. The second proposal is perhaps less radical: that LRECs should be majority-lay (as in Denmark).

One justification for the first proposal is this: the role of LRECs is unacceptably paternalistic as it currently stands. On the one hand, their right to veto research on the grounds that it cannot achieve its end may be a valuable contribution. On the other hand, their right to veto it on the grounds that it has no valuable end or is too risky to take part in, is an infringement of the liberty of individuals to decide what they want to do. For instance, it could be argued that the decision to make a bold gesture of moral altruism in volunteering for a study of possibly very harmful yet potentially hugely beneficial new developments, should be left to individuals.

A number of things may be said in response. Just one will be considered here. Someone may argue that, in some cases, simply asking someone to take part in research constitutes a pressure to do so, or may cause harm. For instance, asking someone if they would be prepared to answer questions relating to the death of a loved one may itself be enough to reawaken memories the person would rather let rest. But, in such cases, the prospective research subjects cannot protect themselves, since the harm occurs in the course of seeking consent. So, seeking the consent of prospective subjects is not enough to ensure that harm unacceptable to them is not done. Ensuring such harm is not done is significant work requiring a veto.

Here, perhaps, the majority-lay committee proposal comes into its own. If subject consent is not a sufficient protection, but subject protection is supposed to be the committee's main interest, why not have a committee which is made up of those who are most likely to have that interest at heart: a committee dominated by lay members. The majority-lay committee could co-opt experts in nursing, medical, statistical and pharmacological, matters, where it lacked these, to act as advisers, giving facts and explaining things. (Co-option already happens in the UK; and in Denmark, where committees are small and have a majority-lay membership by law, lack of expertise is part remedied in this way (Holm, 1992, p. 11).)

Lay power of this sort has precedents, in the jury system, for example. Holm, pointing out the lay dominance of the Danish system, also reports that this did not seem to have threatened the standards of review (Holm, 1992, pp. 9–11). What might be the objection to such a lay dominance on a gatekeeping LREC in the UK? One practical argument might be that, unless membership itself is to be increased, a lay-dominated REC would have perhaps only five professional health carers on it. Thus, co-option of expertise might have to increase, which might present logistical difficulties. Practical objections have a moral aspect, in that practical problems may slow up review, which might mean unnecessary delay to the start of good research. An increase of membership numbers may not be seen as desirable from this point of view either.

However, someone may argue that there must be a limit to how far appeals to delay and logistics may go.

Conclusion

The limit which may be in someone's mind is that implied in the Declaration of Helsinki, and quoted earlier, that "in research on man, the interest of science and society should never take precedence over considerations related to the wellbeing of the subject". Ethical review, being a step in the research process, of necessity holds up research. The justification for this hold-up lies (in part) in the distinctiveness of attitude which may be taken towards these primary considerations by a genuinely independent review. Many good reasons may be given for quickly starting a research project involving human subjects. But, it may be argued that these do not, and should not, override the duty of society, the NHS, the researchers and their sponsors, and indeed of the LREC itself, to ensure that independent review is carried out for the protection of the potential research subjects.

Acknowledgements

I would very much like to thank Louise de Raeve and Don Evans for their helpful comments and suggestions.

References

Armstrong, M. (1988) *Ethics – A Nursing Viewpoint*. Institute of Medical Ethics Bulletin Supplement No. 8. London: Institute of Medical Ethics.

Beecher, H. (1966) Ethics and clinical research. *New England Journal of Medicine,* **274,** 1354.

Benster, R. and Pollock, A. (1992) Ethics and multicentre research. *British Medical Journal,* **304,** 1696.

Bergkamp, L. (1988) American IRBs and Dutch research ethics committees: how they compare. *IRB: A Review of Human Subjects Research,* **10** (Sept.–Oct.), 1.

Byrne, P. (1988) Medical research and the human subject: problems of consent and control in the UK experience. *Annals of the New York Academy of Science,* **530,** 144.

Clothier Committee (1992) *Report of the Committee on the Ethics of Gene Therapy.* CM 1788. London: HMSO.

Department of Health (1991) *Local Research Ethics Committees.* London: Department of Health.

Department of Health and Human Services (1981) 45 CFR.

Department of Health and Social Security (1975) Supervision of the Ethics of Clinical Research Investigations and Fetal Research. HSC(IS)153.

Department of Health Education and Welfare (1974) 45 CFR 46.

Doyal, L. (1994) Towards a standard application form for LRECs. *Bulletin of Medical Ethics,* **101** (September), 15.

Drury, M. (1992) Ethics and multicentre research. *British Medical Journal,* **304,** 1696.

Evans, D. (1992a) Report to the Department of Health on the Conduct of Ethical Review of Multi-Location Research Involving Human Subjects.

Evans, D. (1992b) Report to the Department of Health on the Training of Local Research Ethics Committees.

Evans, D., Evans, M., Greaves, D. and Morgan, D. (1992) *Trainers' Manual for the Training of Members of Research Ethics Committees.*

Faulder, C. (1985) *Whose Body is it?* London: Virago Press.

Herman, S. (1989) A noninstitutional review board comes of age. *IRB: A Review of Human Subjects Research,* **11** (March–April), 1.

Holm, S. (1992) How many lay members can you have in your IRB? – an overview of the Danish system. *IRB: A Review of Human Subjects Research,* **14** (Nov.–Dec.), 8.

Jacox, A. (1980) Nursing's statement: testifying in Washington. In Davis, A. and Krueger, J. (eds) *Patients, Nurses, Ethics.* New York: American Journal of Nursing Co.

Levine, R. (1986) *Ethics and Regulation of Clinical Research,* second edition. Baltimore and Munich: Urban and Schwarzenberg.

Levine, R. (1988) Protection of human subjects of biomedical research in the United States. A contrast with recent experience in the United Kingdom. *Annals of the New York Academy of Sciences,* **530,** 133.

Medicines Control Agency (1995) *The Medicines For Human Use (Marketing Authorisations etc.) Regulations 1994. S.I. 1994/3144.* London: Medicines Control Agency Information Centre.

Moodie, P. and Marshall, T. (1992) Guidelines for local research ethics committees. *British Medical Journal*, **304**, 1293.

National Commission for the Protection of Human Subjects of Biomedical and Behavioral Research (1978) *Institutional Review Boards: Report and Recommendations.* Washington, DC: Department of Health Education and Welfare (DHEW) publication no. (OS) 78-0008. Appendix, DHEW publication no. (OS) 78-0009.

Nicholson, R. (ed.) (1986) *Medical Research With Children: Ethics, Law, and Practice.* The Report of an Institute of Medical Ethics working group on the ethics of clinical research investigations on children. Oxford: Oxford University Press.

Nuremberg Military Tribunals (1949) Nuremberg Code ("Permissible Medical Experiments"). In *Trials of War Criminals before the Nuernberg Military Tribunals under Control Council Law No. 10: Nuernberg, October 1946–April 1949*, Vol. 2, p. 181. Washington: US Government Printing Office (n.d.).

Pelerin, M. and Hall, S. (1992) Ethics and multicentre research. *British Medical Journal*, **304**, 1696.

Polkinghorn Committee (1989) *Review of the Guidance on the Research Use of Fetuses and Fetal Material ("The Polkinghorn Report").* CM 762. London: HMSO.

Royal College of Nursing (1977) *Ethics Related to Research in Nursing.* London: Royal College of Nursing.

Royal College of Nursing Research Advisory Group (1993) *Ethics Related to Research in Nursing.* London: Royal College of Nursing.

Royal College of Physicians Committee on the Supervision of the Ethics of Clinical Investigations in Institutions (1967) *Report.* London: RCP.

Royal College of Physicians Committee on the Supervision of the Ethics of Clinical Research Investigations in Institutions (1973) *Report.* London: RCP.

Taskforce on the Strategy for Research in Nursing, Midwifery and Health Visiting (1993) *Report.* Department of Health.

Welsh National Board for Nursing Midwifery and Health Visiting (1991) *The Development of Critical Awareness – An Advisory Paper.*

12

Teaching Nursing and Midwifery Research

Donna Mead

The central theme of this chapter will focus on the tensions which exist when patients/clients are used as research subjects by nurses and midwives who are in the process of learning about research. Clinical areas have been saturated by neophyte researchers undertaking very small studies in part fulfilment of course requirements. An analysis of why this has happened will be developed and, in particular, the ethical issues of using the general public as research subjects by students will be explored. The importance of ensuring that research training exists will be acknowledged. Several ways of achieving this while protecting the public will be described.

Whenever research ethics are taught to students certain topics are thoroughly covered. These include human rights, informed consent, the role of local research ethics committees and so on. At the centre of this teaching is that the patient/client should be protected from harm. Concepts such as confidentiality and anonymity, therefore, are covered well. Teachers are aware that patients tend to be captive and submissive audiences who may fear reprisals if they decline to participate in research, so they go to great lengths to ensure that students understand the consequence of such fears which can influence patients into agreeing to participate when they would rather not. Students are taught to ensure that the patient understands the identity of the person doing the research, i.e. that when a nurse, midwife or doctor requests a patient to participate in a study, at that moment they are "researcher" first and clinician second and that patients need to put aside images of good nurse or doctor (who will do them no harm and act as their advocate) for one of "scientist". Paradoxically, by allowing students, in particular pre-registration students, to undertake research on patients/clients we may be at risk of violating many of these principles.

The 1972 Committee on nursing stated that nursing should become a research based profession and that: "a sense of the need for research should become part of the mental equipment for every practising nurse or midwife". Since then, research has become a central feature of most curricula. Initially, this began as an awareness, understanding and appreciation of nursing research. Latterly, this has come to include an opportunity for students to undertake a piece of research. Several individuals have called for this practice to be discontinued (James, 1990; Neuberger, 1991; WNB, 1991; Coleman and Mead, 1993). This is because many tensions arise when patients/clients are used as research subjects by nurses and midwives who are in the process of learning about research. Most of the ethical issues arise because problems stem from research being used as an educational tool. James (1990) attributed these to the sheer volume and level of skill of those trying to obtain access to patients which created both practical and ethical issues.

Sheer Volume

The numbers of students (nursing, medical and paramedical) who wanted to gain access to patients and clients in order to undertake small-scale research in part fulfilment of a course of study was staggering. This included pre-registration students, post-basic students, undergraduate and post-graduate students. It was felt that there was a danger of such research over-saturating clinical areas. This was seen to compromise the chances of the serious researcher being given access. More importantly though, it was felt that educationalists had lost sight of the need to protect patients' rights to our care by not recognising the difference between the imperative of care and the imperative of research (Regional Representatives on Nursing Research, 1989). The question which needed to be asked was: "What are the students trying to access and is it appropriate?" Is it appropriate in terms of the numbers involved? If this was the only concern then it could be resolved by reducing the numbers of students doing research. Appropriateness is linked, too, with concerns about the level of skill of the students undertaking this research. Incidentally, as a result of the NHS reforms, there has been a huge increase in the amount of audit activities carried out. The processes involved in audit are, in many ways, identical to those of research (except that ethical permission is not required in order to carry out audit). This again adds to the sheer volume of individuals approaching patients to collect data.

Level of Skill

Students were trying to gain access to vulnerable individuals who needed nursing or midwifery care, in order to undertake a process, namely research, which was not necessary as part of that care. Neuberger (1991) felt that sick people should not be subjected to research which was a requirement of a student's training. She said that research can be invasive, posing questions about pain, risk and benefit but it can also be emotionally threatening, with questions which are too personal. In fact Faulkner (1980) argued that even a simple, anonymous questionnaire was an invasion of privacy. Of course an invasion of privacy may be justified if the outcome is the generation of knowledge which has the possibility of being used to benefit others. It is doubtful that this was the case for several reasons.

Knowledge Generation

(1) The main reason for the research being undertaken was to enable the students to learn research skills and to provide them with a qualification.

(2) There is usually a short period of time to complete research which is part of a course. Consequently, research designs are often compromised and the research tends to be small in scale. What is feasible in the time allowed is likely to have more of an influence on design than scientific criteria. A longitudinal design may be the most appropriate but, with insufficient time for this, a compromise is made. A cross-section may be used or post-test/intervention data collected too early. This has been the case, for example, with research in the field of primary nursing (Mead, 1993) with post-implementation data being collected before the staff had sufficient time to fully implement new patterns of working. Inevitably, the results of such research are flawed and the "knowledge" generated is criticised because of these weaknesses.

(3) In order for research to benefit future patients, the findings have to be disseminated to the profession. However, few, if any, student projects find their way into the literature. If they were to be submitted (and few are) then many of them would be rejected because of methodological weakness (size and type of sample, for example). These methodological weaknesses are likely to be the result of either the students' lack of skill or insufficient time being allowed for the most appropriate design.

(4) To overcome the difficulties associated with time and level of skills, students are sometimes advised to do a replication study. The findings obtained may contribute to a body of knowledge, but these may not be as directly applicable as they were to the first research area or they may be applicable in a much more limited way, e.g. to a single ward.

It could be argued that each student is allocated a supervisor whose role it is to oversee the research process and that this resembles what happens when students go on a placement to learn clinical skills. There, students are usually allocated a mentor whose responsibility it is to facilitate and supervise learn-ing. When the mentor is not there, others are present who can supervise and, should problems arise, there is a qualified nurse available to assist. The research supervisor is not usually present when data are being collected. Even though the research supervisor may train the student in these techniques, they would not be at hand when they were being carried out with patients/clients. It may be the case that no one else on the ward or in the community team is skilled in research either.

There are many examples where this situation has caused harm. For ex-ample, six women who had received a mastectomy were interviewed three days post-operatively by a pre-registration student nurse who was interested in the problems the women thought they might have with sexuality. The women were being cared for on the ward where the student was undertaking her clinical placement. One person informed the student that her main fears were not about sexuality but about having cancer and the possibility of dying from it. This was recorded as part of the research data but not dealt with. The student who understood about confidentiality in research felt that it was inappropriate to pass this information on. There are several lessons to be learned from this.

A skilled clinician and researcher would be able to deal with the woman's actual fears. The imperative of care may lead to the clinician deciding that, in this instance, the woman should be excluded from the research because it is more important to deal with her fears than to carry on with the research process. The researcher would realise that because the woman had just voiced these fears, her mind was more likely to be on these than sexuality (the topic of the research) and that any data collected at this time would be contaminated by this fact.

When the woman concerned told her husband about what had happened, a complaint was made, which was how the situation was discovered. This research should not have been allowed because it was unsound methodo-logically and ethically (interviewing women at this time) and the local re-search ethics committee should have rejected it. After all, a brief interview with six women is not going to result in new knowledge. These concerns are part of the problem. Not all small projects are put to the local research ethics committee. Neuberger (1991) noted that LRECs have no powers to force researchers to clear proposals with them. There are those who think that very small studies which are being carried out as part of a scheme of study do not require ethical clearance as their status is the same as any student project, for example a care study, for which ethical approval is not sought. However, it can be seen that this was an unethical study, first of all because bad research is unethical research and, secondly, because the expected benefits from it were not likely to justify the demands made on the human subjects involved.

Clearly, it should not have been passed by the student's supervisor, but this raises another area of concern. As the numbers of courses requiring students to carry out research increased at such an alarming rate, there simply were not sufficient nurse teachers with the skills to supervise them adequately. This situation should never have arisen for if one looks at course requirements then, "undertaking" a piece of research was not a criterion.

Prior to Project 2000 the competencies for nurses are found in Rule 18 of Statutory Instrument 1983 No. 873 (The Nurses, Midwives and Health Visitors Rule Approval Order 1983), while the competencies for Project 2000 courses are contained in an amendment to Statutory Instrument 1983 No. 873, Statutory Instrument 1989 No. 1456 (The Nurses, Midwives and Health Visitors Registered Fever Nurses Amendment Rules and Training Amendment Rules Approval Order 1989), which inserts a new rule 18. The new rule 18 makes no mention of research but it is clear that, in order to achieve competencies, and to continue to remain competent, individuals would have to be aware of research findings and appreciate the importance of research in the development of practice. Rule 18a makes explicit reference to the "use" of relevant literature and research to inform the practice of nursing.

Many of the issues which have been discussed above apply to both qualified and unqualified staff. For both groups the common problem is that knowledge generation is neither the aim nor a realistic possibility when the objective is to learn about research. Where the qualified nurse is carrying out a small study as part of a course requirement, then it would be difficult to justify the research for ethical reasons. Here, too, there is no statutory requirement for a piece of research to be carried out. Health Visitor Training Rules are set out in Part IV of the Statutory Instrument, while outcomes for midwifery education are set out in Rule 33 of Statutory Instrument 1990 No 1624 (The Nurses, Midwives and Health Visitors [Midwife training] Amendment Rules Approval Order 1990). The outcomes for midwifery education make reference to the "use" of relevant literature and research to inform the practice of midwifery.

None of these sets of competencies or learning outcomes includes a requirement that the practitioner should be competent to undertake original research. It is sufficient that practitioners should be knowledgeable about the research which exists (relevant to their practice speciality) that they should be able to evaluate research reports critically and should understand the need, where appropriate, to modify practice in the light of research. The skills which are required, therefore, include critical awareness, analysis, synthesis and informed decision making (WNB, 1991).

There are many more courses, however, than those which lead to a statutory qualification. The continuing education framework set up under the auspices of the National Boards in England and Wales, for example, have a number of short post-basic courses. In the past many of these required that the student carry out a small research project. In 1991 the Welsh National Board put out the following in an advisory paper:

> the learning outcomes for current Welsh National Board courses do not require the skills of a researcher, and the Board does not believe that students should engage in projects involving the collection of data from human subjects unless the learning outcomes for the course explicitly require the development of such skills . . . The ability to review critically a body of literature, analyse the information and arguments found therein, and to come to a judgement on the basis of this exercise, involves higher order intellectual skills and, it could be argued the way to teach and develop such skills is through reading, debate and discussion and the writing of reviews (WNB, 1991).

This position is one which is welcomed. However, the paper is advisory and does allow that certain courses may explicitly require the development of research skills. Nevertheless, this is an indication that the trend is reversing because the profession has realised the ethical implications involved in carrying out very small research projects on human subjects.

Teaching Research Ethics to Graduate Studies Students

What is the situation when nurses and midwives are studying for a degree? In the UK there are two types of undergraduate student. Those who read for a Bachelor's degree as part of initial nurse training and trained nurses who are studying for a degree (usually a part-time scheme of study). There are two types of degree at Master's level. The first is a taught course and would normally have two components to the examination, one of which would include a small research study. The second type is a research degree and typically leads to the award of the degree of Master of Philosophy. Finally, there are doctoral degrees. There are several types. The first is called the degree of Doctor of Philosophy and is referred to as either Ph.D. or D. Phil.; the second is a taught degree which includes a research component (there are very few of these in the UK currently, although they are quite common in the USA). Finally, there is a doctor's degree which is awarded on the basis of personal contribution to scholarship in a field. All the individual's papers and research reports are reviewed and the degree may be awarded if these are considered to have made an outstanding contribution to knowledge in the field. Does a case exist for students studying for one of these degrees to be allowed access to patients to undertake research? In order to answer this question, the need to undertake research and the type of research has to be compared with the outcome criteria for these schemes of study.

Research Degrees

Doctoral degrees (by research)

The generation of new knowledge is a criteria for study at doctoral level. This will require original research of appropriate scope. The use of human subjects can be justified because new knowledge will result which has the potential to benefit others.

The degree of Magister (by research)

For the degree of Master of Philosophy, the generation of new knowledge may not be the result. The student may be required to build on what is already known. Alternatively, the student may need to work in a new field, one for which knowledge does not exist. Access to human subjects may be necessary and justifiable, ethically, for research at this level also.

Both of the above schemes of study are regarded as research training. However, the time devoted to these schemes allows for appropriate training in both method and the ethical and moral issues of research.

The degree of Magister (by examination and thesis)

The objective in courses of study at taught master's level is that students should be able to demonstrate an understanding of the research process and an ability to locate and critically analyse appropriate literature. These students would be required to demonstrate that they have built on the sum of what is known in a field by developing the thinking and arguments which pertain. New knowledge is not a criteria for success for study at this level. For the student of a taught master's course, however, competence in carrying out a piece of research may be a criterion. In other words, it may be seen as research training only. It will be expected that following completion of a taught master's course, an individual will be competent to carry out research, albeit with supervision. Such an individual will need to experience the research process.

The degree of Bachelor

The student who is studying for a bachelor's degree as part of initial nurse training is no different from any other pre-registration student (they are neither a competent clinician nor researcher). It is not necessary for such a student to carry out research which involves human subjects. The qualified nurse who is reading for a bachelor's degree is a competent clinician but not a competent researcher.

It has been argued that, for research degrees, it is necessary to carry out research which may involve human subjects. Since the research will be of sufficient scope and the findings have the potential to generate new knowledge and/or to benefit others, the use of human subjects can be justified. At taught master's level, there may be alternatives to using human subjects while still meeting the criteria for the course and enabling research training to take place. At bachelor's level and for post-basic courses generally, the use of human subjects cannot be justified.

If this position is accepted, it would not bode well for the future. As a result of the move into higher education, all nursing departments must generate good-quality research. They will be assessed on the contribution made to research. Their funding and likelihood to attract students will depend on this. Also it is via Project 2000 (undergraduate in particular) that the future foundations of nursing research will be strengthened. If nursing is to develop its knowledge base, it is vital that education in the critical appreciation of research is provided and that staff are trained in research. It will not be desirable in the future to leave research to the academics. The NHS reforms have ensured this. Commissioners of services will require evidence of research-based care (through research-based clinical guidelines); providers of care will want to demonstrate that they are evaluating the effectiveness of care given. The skills which are necessary to do this are learned by doing research. For this to happen there will need to be a *critical mass* of research-competent nurses in practice. Having such a critical mass will mean that there are sufficient numbers of nurses who are skilled in undertaking and critically appraising research and in implementing findings. The problem is that the number of nurses studying for research degrees is very small. We would never achieve this critical mass if we relied solely on those undertaking the courses in which access to human subjects would be allowed. We cannot avoid the position, though, that it is research as an educational tool which creates the biggest problem ethically.

The next section focuses on ways of ensuring that students can experience the research process, and so develop the appropriate skills, and be able to do this without having access to patients and clients. Some of the methodological issues are presented in a lot of detail. This is done in order to demonstrate how much can be learned about the research process in this way. The experience can be as rich as if the students had collected the data for themselves. This can be achieved in a number of ways:

(1) use of data banks;
(2) simulation;
(3) use of data which have been collected as part of a research study but not yet analysed;
(4) collection of data which do not involve patients/clients.

Use of Data Banks

The use of data banks for research training is not new. For example the ESRC data archive* at Essex University has been used for the secondary analysis of data. It is a fairly straightforward task to set up such archives in individual departments. Data sets are available from academic staff who carry out research and staff from other universities will often be prepared to make some of their data sets available for this purpose. The first step in the process is to take a data set and "clean it up". This means ensuring that it is anonymised (if it is not already) so that there is no chance that the student will recognise the research respondents/participants. No attempt is made to sanitise the data, so if there are flaws, then these remain. The student would not be told whether the data set being issued was regarded as good or bad. The next step would be to provide, as accompanying material, the research question and a list of the referenced literature which resulted in the question being formulated. The student would be required to locate that literature, update and evaluate it.

If, for example, the research involved interviews as the method of data collection, the interview data can be provided in several ways:

(1) the audiotapes;
(2) the transcripts on a disk in ASCII format;
(3) hard copy of the transcripts;
(4) the transcripts entered into the appropriate software (e.g. Ethnograph, Nudist, Paradox) and ready to analyse.

A choice would be made according to the student and the course involved. The student can comment on whether interviewing was the most appropriate method of data collection and on the conduct of the interview by picking up on leading questions and so on. Experience in transcribing can be gained, if this is thought necessary. If there is time, it is worth allowing the student to experience this. They become immersed in the data and familiar with it as a consequence. This assists in analysis later. They also gain a realistic picture of the sheer hard work and time-consuming nature of this aspect of the research process.

If a questionnaire was the method of data collection, then a similar process can be used. Once again the questionnaires will need to be anonymised. This rarely presents a problem. Questionnaires are usually coded in order to identify the respondent. This code usually takes the form of a series of numerical digits. These codes are necessary to aid the analysis. For example, the first digit may represent a geographical area. If there was a question on "type of surgery preferred" then, if wished, this can be cross-tabulated with geographical area to see if people who live in different parts of the country prefer different types of surgery. It is quite straightforward to devise a second

* Called "Biron". University of Essex, Colchester, Essex CO4 3SQ, UK.

coding framework which means the same as the initial one but which could not lead to identification of the original respondents.

The questionnaires can be provided in several ways:

(1) in hard copy with the responses uncoded;
(2) in hard copy with the responses coded;
(3) on a disk with the responses already entered on to an appropriate soft-ware program (e.g. SPSS PC, EPINFO or MINITAB).

The design of some questionnaires is such that the answers have to be coded numerically before they can be entered into the computer. More often though it is the case that the questions are pre-coded. For example:

> Is your ward regularly closed at the weekend?
> Please tick yes or no.

yes   no

[ ] 1   [ ] 2

12

The figure 12 refers to the code which will need to be entered before the code 1 or 2 depending on whether the respondent ticks yes or no. This is so that the question will be recognised by the statistical package used. Using this format will speed up the data entry process and increase the likelihood of accuracy.

A student who is given an uncoded questionnaire learns much about coding and, more importantly, becomes immersed in the data in much the same way as the student who is given audiotapes to transcribe. There may have been problems with the design of certain questions. These cause problems which the student can identify. For example:

> What is your age?
>
> Please tick on box   ✔
>
> 15–20 years   [ ]
>
> 20–25 years   [ ]
>
> 25–30 years   [ ]
>
> 30–35 years   [ ]

A student presented with such a questionnaire in order to enter data and analyse it will soon pick up on the problems of respondents being able to tick more than one box if aged 20, 25 or 30.

One of the purposes of questionnaires is to look for relationships between variables. For example, a school careers teacher may send out a questionnaire on career choices. There may be questions on sex and A level subjects and career preferences. By cross-tabulating the variables, he may find that boys who take science subjects are unlikely to select nursing as a career choice. He may wish to advise such pupils that nursing should be considered. The student of research would not know what cross-tabulations had been performed initially and may decide to look for relationships which the original researcher did not do. In one such instance the student researcher decided to cross-tabulate the choice of A-level subjects with the career choices indicated. He found that many students who indicated nursing as career preference were taking the wrong mix of A-level subjects (Art, Art & Design, English). This would lead to them being refused admission to university courses and at a time when it would be too late to alter the subjects. The schoolteacher who had given his data set for analysis by students learning about research was informed about this and his career advice changed accordingly. Thus, not only did the student learn about research but he was able also to contribute to the sum of what was known about the issue of career choices.

Simulation

There are several ways in which the teacher of research can provide research simulation. The approach involves providing data sets based on questionnaires which the students have designed or on interviews which they have conducted. In either case the student would identify the topic to be studied, locate and review the appropriate literature, define the research question and choose an appropriate research design.

If the appropriate research design is a questionnaire, then the student would go on to design one. Having then decided on the size and type of sample (which can be anything from ten to tens of thousands; there is no difference in the amount of effort involved) the questionnaire is then handed to the teacher who subsequently provides the student with a data set generated from the questionnaire. Step-by-step instructions on how this is done can be found in Coleman and Mead (1993). However, a software package such as EPI INFO (Dean *et al.*, 1990) can be used. This has a facility to create data sets for teaching purposes. Any tables produced can be imported into other commonly used statistical packages. EPI INFO is public domain software and is available free of charge. If the teacher notices questions which would in a real situation lead to flawed results, then the data can be manipulated so that this shows up. In this way, the student learns meaningfully from their mistakes.

If an interview is the appropriate method, then students can carry these out on each other. Guidance at the outset is essential in this instance so that topics which other students would have knowledge or experience of are chosen. For example, a group of taught master's students comprised educators (nursing and midwifery) and experienced clinicians. As Project 2000 was about to start, all of them had been grappling with the issue of mentorship.

It was decided to use this as a topic for both the interview and question-naire. Some students conducted the interviews among the groups, others were involved in the design of a questionnaire which the whole group filled in. There were two distinct groups in the sample; educators and clinicians. What emerged was a shared understanding of definitions of mentorship. However, there was a marked distinction in how the two groups thought that mentorship should be carried out in practice. The educators felt that the student should be allocated to a mentor. The clinicians felt that mentorship was something that happened naturally. This became the topic of a lively debate on the issue and, eventually, the topic of a research study. Those who conducted the interviews experienced the problems associated with this method (for example, that from a five minute interview, a huge number of data are generated; some students had allowed their colleagues to talk for 40 minutes). From this they learned the lessons of appropriate sample size and interview length.

Use of Data which Have been Collected as Part of a Research Study but Not Yet Analysed

It is usually the case with most research studies that, at the end, some of the data are not analysed. This is not because people set out knowingly to collect data which will not be used. Sometimes relationships in the data become apparent but there may not be time to investigate them or to do so would detract from the main theme of the research. Nevertheless, these relationships are worth exploring at a later date. I do not mean data dredging which means that one explores the data for every possible aspect of analysis simply because they are there. Research is a dynamic process, and sometimes links occur that were not planned for in the design. If they were to be investigated, however, they might add considerably to the sum of what is known in a field.

For example, in one study the ward sisters were asked to list the five most important jobs which they undertook each day, together with the one which they would be most reluctant to give up. The intention was to note the extent to which activities commensurate with primary nursing were mentioned. This could then be correlated with the extent to which primary nursing was claimed to be practised. In this way it acted as a consistency check. It became apparent that these data would give an approximation of each ward sister's management style and that as well as correlating this with the incidence of primary nursing overall, it could be correlated ward by ward. An analysis of ward sisters' management styles was not the intention of the original research. The question was included as a consistency check, an indication of validity. This analysis was not, therefore, performed at the time of the original research. It would have detracted from the research plan and led to delays in completion. However, this project was later given to a student of research who learned much about the research process as a result, including the need to be on the look-out for serendipitous opportunities to discover more about a topic.

Collection of Data which Do Not Involve Patients and Clients

The inventive teacher can find many ways that will enable the student to collect data and experience each stage of the research process without using patients. This may include problem-solving activities. For example, a ward sister may be concerned about the difficulties in organising the off-duty rota so that a primary or associate nurse can be available to care for a patient at any given time. The tension is well known. The sister needs to be sure that each day there is an appropriate mix of staff to cater for admissions, operating lists, consultants' rounds as well as the needs of individual patients and nurses. In this instance the student could conduct a literature review to discover how common this problem is and whether there are any solutions. If one seemed appropriate then this could be introduced and evaluated. This could not be regarded as research *per se*. However, the student would learn much about the research process as a consequence and, of course, would be acting ethically.

It may be possible to look at other practices. For instance, one undergraduate student who was already a registered nurse thought that the menu on the children's ward on which she worked was inappropriate. The food was enticing for the children, for example chips, sausages and beefburgers as a regular feature. Thus the children would eat the food but the diet was not balanced. A process of inquiry began. It was discovered that the catering staff had been concerned about the amount of food which was returned to the kitchen uneaten. That had resulted in an inappropriate menu. A literature review was conducted. Had anyone else reported this pattern and if so what had they done about it? The dietitian, nurse and catering staff modified the diet. The image was improved with cartoon characters eating wholesome food depicted on the menu cards. A mix of wholesome and "popular" food was provided and instead of sending the food up from the kitchen plated for each child, a selection of foods in containers was delivered and the nurses chose from these. The student collected data on the amount of food wasted by looking at the amount of food returned. This problem-solving approach mirrored the research process and did not involve patients directly.

A nurse who was interested in complementary therapies read a paper in one of the nursing journals which said that many of these practices contravene Judaeo-Christian beliefs. This came as a surprise. The number of complementary therapies is vast, as was discovered from the literature review. The student decided to develop a taxonomy of these practices which was based on place of origin, underlying beliefs, type of intervention and so on. When a taxonomy which held together logically was devised, the Bible was used as a theoretical framework from which to evaluate the practices contained in each of the categories in the taxonomy. Some, but not all, were found to be unsound biblically. This provided an important contribution to knowledge in the field. The attention to detail which is required when developing a taxonomy mirrors the research process. The results will be helpful to practitioners and no patients were involved.

Sometimes students collect data which have nothing to do with nursing or health care *per se*. This does not matter if the objective is to learn about research. One student decided to look at the register for marriages at her local church. Entries for the last 100 years were examined. A literature review about local industry and important events during the time period was undertaken. It was then possible to look at the employment pattern, age on getting married, etc. and to compare these in periods of 25 years. Thus the student learned much about her own community. The process is one which mirrors epidemiological research.

These are a few of many examples. One note of caution is necessary. It may be possible to conduct research or to undertake problem-solving activities which do not involve patients. If these are carried out within the NHS, it may still be desirable to put the research design before the local research ethics committee for approval.

All of these examples demonstrate that it is possible to provide a rich and meaningful experience for students who need to learn about research while not involving patients. In many cases this results in an addition to the sum of what is know about a topic. This is the *raison d'être* for any research study. It can also be seen that experience in both research traditions (positivist and interpretive) can be gained in the methods which have been outlined. It would be misleading not to acknowledge that many students will feel disappointed if they cannot do the project that they want. Many students want to take the opportunity to investigate something which has intrigued them for years or to look at an issue which they feel passionately about. This has to be handled sensitively. The appropriate teaching of research ethics will assist in this. The way in which the alternatives are presented has to suggest a meaningful and rich experience for the student. Students can be convinced that if the issue they want to research is so important, it would be better for them to learn the appropriate skills first. Then they can carry out the research which they really want to do. So many research studies undertaken as the student's first research encounter end up with a limitation section stating that the student's inexperience contributed to a number of flaws, thus diminishing confidence in the results.

Students who have used the methods described are usually satisfied, even if some persuasion was necessary initially. Some empirical work would increase the confidence in this conclusion. The time allowed for the research project in some schemes of study is so short that an intolerable burden is placed on the student who has to gain approval from ethical committees, which can take a long time to process proposals. When this is the case, the objectives of the course team have to be questioned. Most students involved in the methods described here say that they feel prepared to carry out research. This surely was always the main objective and it has been achieved ethically.

References

Coleman, M. and Mead, D.M. (1993) Simulation in training questionnaire design. *Nurse Researcher*, **1**(2), 52–61.

Dean, A., Dean, J., Burton, A. and Dicker, R. (1990) *EPI INFO, Version 5, A Word Processing, Database and Statistics Program for Epidemiology on Microcomputers*. Stone Mountain, GA: USD Incorporated.

Faulkner, A. (1980) Nursing as a research based profession: some ethical issues. *Nursing Focus*, August, 476–481.

James, N. (1990) Nursing research in Wales: conundrum or tension of stratification and change? Paper presented to the Welsh Senior Nurse Colloquium, Llandrindod Wells, March.

Mead, D.M. (1993) The development of primary nursing in N.H.S. care giving institutions in Wales. Unpublished Ph.D. thesis, University of Wales.

Neuberger, J. (1991) *Ethics and Health Care: the Role of Research Ethics Committees in the UK*. Research Report 13. London: King's Fund Institute.

WNB (1991) The development of critical awareness – an advisory paper. Welsh National Board for Nursing, Midwifery and Health Visiting.

Appendix

World Medical Association Declaration of Helsinki.

Recommendations guiding physicians in biomedical research involving human subjects

Adopted by the 18th World Medical Assembly, Helsinki, Finland, June 1964 and amended by the 29th World Medical Assembly, Tokyo, Japan, October 1975, 35th World Medical Assembly, Venice, Italy, October 1983 and the 41st World Medical Assembly, Hong Kong, September 1989

Introduction

It is the mission of the physician to safeguard the health of the people. His or her knowledge and conscience are dedicated to the fulfillment of this mission.

The Declaration of Geneva of the World Medical Association binds the physician with the words, "The Health of my patient will be my first consideration", and the International Code of Medical Ethics declares that "A physician shall act only in the patient's interest when providing medical care which might have the effect of weakening the physical and mental condition of the patient."

The purpose of biomedical research involving human subjects must be to improve diagnostic, therapeutic and prophylactic procedures and the understanding of the aetiology and pathogenesis of disease.

In current medical practice most diagnostic, therapeutic or prophylactic procedures involve hazards. This applies especially to biomedical research.

Medical progress is based on research which ultimately must rest in part on experimentation involving human subjects.

In the field of biomedical research a fundamental distinction must be recognised between medical research in which the aim is essentially diagnostic or therapeutic for a patient, and medical research, the essential object of which is purely scientific and without implying direct diagnostic or therapeutic value to the person subjected to the research.

Special caution must be exercised in the conduct of research which may affect the environment, and the welfare of animals used for research must be respected.

Because it is essential that the results of laboratory experiments be applied to human beings to further scientific knowledge and to help suffering humanity, the World Medical Association has prepared the following recommendations as a guide to every physician in biomedical research involving human subjects. They should be kept under review in the future. It must be stressed that the standards as drafted are only a guide to physicians all over the world. Physicians are not relieved from criminal, civil and ethical responsibilities under the laws of their own countries.

I. Basic Principles

(1) Biomedical research involving human subjects must conform to generally accepted scientific principles and should be based on adequately performed laboratory and animal experimentation and on a thorough knowledge of the scientific literature.

(2) The design and performance of each experimental procedure involving human subjects should be clearly formulated in an experimental protocol which should be transmitted for consideration, comment and guidance to a specially appointed committee independent of the investigator and the sponsor provided that this independent committee is in conformity with the laws and regulations of the country in which the research experiment is performed.

(3) Biomedical research involving human subjects should be conducted only by scientifically qualified persons and under the supervision of a clinically copent medical person. The responsibility for the human subject must always rest with a medically qualified person and never rest on the subject of the research, even though the subject has given his or her consent.

(4) Biomedical research involving human subjects cannot legitimately be carried out unless the importance of the objective is in proportion to the inherent risk to the subject.

(5) Every biomedical research project involving human subjects should be

preceded by careful assessment of predictable risks in comparison with foreseeable benefits to the subject or to others. Concern for the interests of the subject must always prevail over the interests of science and society.

(6) The right of the research subject to safeguard his or her integrity must always be respected. Every precaution should be taken to respect the privacy of the subject and to minimize the impact of the study on the subject's physical and mental integrity and on the personality of the subject.

(7) Physicians should abstain from engaging in research projects involving human subjects unless they are satisfied that the hazards involved are believed to be predictable. Physicians should cease any investigation if the hazards are found to outweigh the potential benefits.

(8) In publication of the results of his or her research, the physician is obliged to preserve the accuracy of the results. Reports of experimentation not in accordance with the principles laid down in this Declaration should not be accepted for publication.

(9) In any research on human beings, each potential subject must be adequately informed of the aims, methods, anticipated benefits and potential hazards of the study and the discomfort it may entail. He or she should be informed that he or she is at liberty to abstain from participation in the study and that he or she is free to withdraw his or her consent to participation at any time. The physician should then obtain the subject's freely-given informed consent, preferably in writing.

(10) When obtaining informed consent for the research project the physician should be particularly cautious if the subject is in a dependent relationship to him or her or may consent under duress. In that case the informed consent should be obtained by a physician who is not engaged in the investigation and who is completely independent of this official relationship.

(11) In case of legal incompetence, informed consent should be obtained from the legal guardian in accordance with national legislation. Where physical or mental incapacity makes it impossible to obtain informed consent, or when the subject is a minor, permission from the responsible relative replaces that of the subject in accordance with national legislation.

Whenever the minor child is in fact able to give a consent, the minor's consent must be obtained in addition to the consent of the minor's legal guardian.

(12) The research protocol should always contain a statement of the ethical considerations involved and should indicate that the principles enunciated in the present Declaration are complied with.

II. Medical Research Combined with Professional Care (Clinical Research)

(1) In the treatment of the sick person, the physician must be free to use a new diagnostic and therapeutic measure, if in his or her judgement it offers hope of saving life, re-establishing health or alleviating suffering.

(2) The potential benefits, hazards and discomfort of a new method should be weighed against the advantages of the best current diagnostic and therapeutic methods.

(3) In any medical study, every patient – including those of a control group, if any – should be assured of the best proven diagnostic and therapeutic method.

(4) The refusal of the patient to participate in a study must never interfere with the physician–patient relationship.

(5) If the physician considers it essential not to obtain informed consent, the specific reasons for this proposal should be stated in the experimental protocol for transmission to the independent committee (I, 2).

(6) The physician can combine medical research with professional care, the objective being the acquisition of new medical knowledge, only to the extent that medical research is justified by its potential diagnostic or therapeutic value for the patient.

III. Non-Therapeutic Biomedical Research Involving Human Subjects (Non-Clinical Biomedical Research)

(1) In the purely scientific application of medical research carried out on a human being, it is the duty of the physician to remain the protector of the life and health of that person on whom biomedical research is being carried out.

(2) The subjects should be volunteers – either healthy persons or patients for whom the experimental design is not related to the patient's illness.

(3) The investigator or the investigating team should discontinue the research if in his/her or their judgement it may, if continued, be harmful to the individual.

(4) In research on man, the interest of science and society should never take precedence over considerations related to the well-being of the subject.

Index